LIVING WITH
MULTIPLE
SCLEROSIS

Living with Multiple Sclerosis

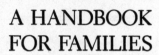

A HANDBOOK FOR FAMILIES

Dr. Robert Shuman and
Dr. Janice Schwartz

Foreword by Robert J. Slater, M.D.

COLLIER BOOKS / MACMILLAN PUBLISHING COMPANY / NEW YORK

MAXWELL MACMILLAN CANADA / TORONTO

MAXWELL MACMILLAN INTERNATIONAL
NEW YORK / OXFORD / SINGAPORE / SYDNEY

Collier Books   Maxwell Macmillan Canada, Inc..
Macmillan Publishing Company   1200 Eglinton Avenue East
866 Third Avenue   Suite 200.
New York, NY 10022   Don Mills, Ontario M3C 3N1

Macmillan Publishing Company is part of the Maxwell Communication
Group of Companies.

Library of Congress Cataloging-in-Publication Data
Shuman, Robert.
[Understanding multiple sclerosis]
Living with multiple sclerosis: a handbook for families / Robert
Shuman and Janice Schwartz.—1st Collier Books ed.
        p.   cm.
Originally published: Understanding multiple sclerosis. New York:
Scribner's, © 1988.
Includes bibliographical references and index.
ISBN 0-02-082026-7
1. Multiple sclerosis—Popular works.   I. Schwartz, Janice.
II. Title.
RC377.S58   1994   93-47116   CIP
362.1'96834—dc20

Macmillan books are available at special discounts for bulk purchases for
sales promotions, premiums, fund-raising, or educational use. For details, contact:

Special Sales Director
Macmillan Publishing Company
866 Third Avenue
New York, NY 10022

First Collier Books Edition 1994

10 9 8 7 6 5 4 3 2 1

Printed in the United States of America

TO

Al, Larry, David,   *Sheila, Rebecca,*
and Susan   *and Daniel*

AND

All of the M.S. families
we have enjoyed working with
through the years.

CONTENTS

FOREWORD

THIS IS A superb collection of experiences, guidelines, questions, and answers that can greatly enhance our day-to-day efforts to deal with disability and achieve a fulfilled and useful life. Although the authors have directed the book specifically at troubles associated with multiple sclerosis, I see it as having broader value, because its lessons deal with issues we all face in daily life. Fear, frustration, anger, denial, feelings of self-worth, relationships with family, friends, employer are things that concern all of us, not just those who have a chronic medical condition. Indeed, for those of us who at the moment are suffering through any of a variety of difficulties, the lessons have direct applicability.

Several dimensions of this book deserve special mention. First, it is eminently readable. The writing style is direct and the concepts clearly set forth. Of particular note is the sensitivity, feeling, even poignancy with which the authors present their thoughts and achieve a discourse that is, at once, both personal and personable.

Second, the chapter themes have been built on issues of everyday life with which we all readily identify: What's happening to me? How do I feel about it? How do you feel? How are we going to work things out? How can I look so well and feel so poorly? How is my memory? Am I thinking straight? What's happened to my sexuality?

A third point is the use of real-life experiences to illustrate specific problems and situations. We identify readily with each of these people. These case analyses provide a professional dimension for the psychological themes under review. In forming the main body of each chapter, they are brief, precise, pithy, and to the point. They "tell the story." Consequently, the book is, likewise, a valuable text for students of psychology and medicine.

The authors have divided the book into three main parts: initial reactions, the adjustment process, and facing the future. Initial reactions are fundamental to all other activities and adjustments. This is borne out by the the authors' elegant handling of the first three chapters, which ask: How am I, the patient, coping with M.S.? How is my spouse or companion? How is my family? Ultimately, the key person in this is the one afflicted, regardless what may be the chronic disease, condition, or disorder. And that person's ability to handle adversity is immensely enhanced by the psychological support of his or her immediate family and circle of friends.

The second chapter, "What Is Happening to You?," sets forth the complexities to be dealt with in our roles as spouses, lovers, and companions, as we are constantly challenged by the ever-present, ever-changing demands of living with chronic illness. This challenge creates the potential for guilt, anger, and unfulfilled expectations among intimate family members and establishes the need—and, in fact, the necessity—to effect what may very well be major changes in their roles regarding friendships, career, and leisure activities. The authors point out with enduring wisdom that there is a difference between life-styles and life values. If we have sound values, they need not change to meet adverse circumstances. Indeed, they provide the anchor to stabilize needed changes in life-styles.

This chapter provides a sensitive portrayal of those life values and emphasizes the importance of the network of shared dependencies and care on which all relationships, marriages, and families are founded. As one woman with M.S. declared, "My husband is my partner, but he is also my best friend." Such a sentiment is the epitome of truly integrated feelings and relationships—and not easily attained!

Chapter 3, on the theme of personal reactions, "What Is Happening to Us?," provides a logical and constructive extension of what family bonding can achieve in aiding and abetting the ability to cope with change. It also depicts the disastrous outcomes of well-meaning or shortsighted responses by both family and patients when inappropriate values dominate behavior. Again, as the authors assert, when a family listens to each other, self-blame, guilt, denial, and anger can be minimized and replaced by positive mutual support.

In this vein, the authors' experiences show that the way a family defines and interprets a serious diagnosis is a major influence on family adjustment. Is it perceived as catastrophic to family integrity, or is it perceived as a challenge to be faced with unifying courage? Again, this reaction is a reflection of the implicit operational family values.

In all of this adaptation and adjustment among the family, there are usually children who must be included in the scenario. They, too, have perceptions that can undergo rapid evolution with changing age. While in their own way they must, and can, carry some of the burden and challenges of family sharing, they can do much to strengthen these bonds and limit their own potential for negative acting-out by early inclusion in the family's adaptation of life-styles to fit life values.

The achievement of other coping strategies dealt with in the remaining chapters flows naturally from the personal relationships depicted at the outset. The transcendental lesson imparted by the authors is that adjustment is complex and continuing, that coping is not easy, and that both must be worked at on the long term. They are, therefore, best confronted early in the course of events by seeking professional consultation from experienced therapists. So much is at stake; so much disaster that can be avoided; so much possibility for a lifetime of rich, enduring experiences.

ROBERT J. SLATER, M.D.
Vice President, Medical Programs,
National Multiple Sclerosis Society, 1977–87
Director, Program on Biomedical Ethics,
National Health Council

ACKNOWLEDGMENTS

WE ARE ESPECIALLY GRATEFUL to Alvan R. Schwartz, M.D., who researched and wrote chapter 12 of this book. Dr. Schwartz's medical knowledge and clinical experience was generously shared with us throughout our writing. He was always available to confirm our descriptions of the medical symptoms of multiple sclerosis.

We also thank: Robert Slater, M.D., of the National Multiple Sclerosis Society and presently director of the National Health Council Incorporated, for his generous foreword and early strong support of this project; Cynthia Zagieboylo, director of support services, and Debra Frankel, special projects manager, both of the Massachusetts chapter of the National Multiple Sclerosis Society, for their time, encouragement, and knowledge of national resources for M.S. persons and their families; June Rollins, for her efficient and forever-cheerful secretarial assistance; and our editor at Scribners, Carrie Chase, for helping to keep the book on track to deadline.

A special thank you to our wonderful agent, Abigail Thomas of the Liz Darhansoff Agency, for her enthusiasm, encouragement, and perseverance about this project.

INTRODUCTION

THERE IS PAIN in living, and sickness and uncertainty. It is the lot of all people to face these facts of life. People with multiple sclerosis and their loved ones may confront adversity earlier and, perhaps, more poignantly than others. But they are not new facts, and we are not alone in having problems, sometimes grave ones, in living. Job in his tent, Buddha beyond his palace gates, and unknown individuals in all times and places have grappled with the challenge of suffering.

The stages of adjustment to chronic illness do not lead in the best cases to a bland acceptance of one's fate. Instead they describe a series of steps of confronting reality more and more directly. At each step we struggle to tear aside a veil that prevents us from acknowledging our position and deciding how, given our circumstances, we are to live. For *that* is the real problem of our lives regardless of health or illness, poverty or wealth.

How am I to live? As psychologists we cannot claim any special answers to this question. What we can do is share with you how people and families with multiple sclerosis have responded. And because one of us has multiple sclerosis and both of us have worked with a great many people with multiple sclerosis, we can offer some insights that you may find useful in coming to the best of terms with the challenge of this illness.

For example, people with multiple sclerosis are often told to "avoid stress." This direction is, of course, doubly humorous. First, because living with multiple sclerosis is itself stressful, and second, because for many people life without stress is life unlived. A widely used rating scale for stress of life events is largely drawn from the ordinary—an argument with a spouse, vacation plans—or the uncontrollable—the death of a spouse, the sickness of a child. How wonderful it might be if we could avoid the stress of either.

And how often those of us with multiple sclerosis get called "stubborn" because we insist on doing chores and taking pleasures that tire us. What others may not realize is how important it is to us to refuse to give up any activity until we have no choice. "If I give this up without a fight, what will go next time without a whimper?" Pride is the term that many people with multiple sclerosis use to refer to their need to do as much as they can as long as they can, regardless of the opinion of loving helpers.

But there is another side to the issue. The woman who continues to do the grocery shopping when her husband has offered to take over the task; the man who continues to mow the lawn despite the affordability of hiring lawn care—each of these may be people who identify what they do, their activities, with who they are.

If she were to ease her stubbornness and he to soften his pride, they might each discover that he or she is more than what one does. The ability to create and sustain relationships, provide good counsel to friends, observe and enjoy nature, read, and expand one's knowledge of the world—all these provide opportunities to *be* more while doing less.

And, of course, with a potentially progressive illness we can put enormous pressure on ourselves to live each day as fully as we can. Yet the decline of physical vigor and mental sharpness is what most of us face regardless of our health. The attempt to live every day as if it is your last may be an unrealistic and unnecessary burden. How often, for example, we tell our children to try their best. But how many of us could keep up such an effort? Perhaps it is better to simply live without worrying about how we or others judge ourselves. It could be that goofing off, wasting time, doing nothing, or fooling around *is* just what the doctor ordered: "Consider the lilies of the field."

In the pages that follow you will meet many people who have been diagnosed with multiple sclerosis. You will learn about their initial reactions, adjustments, denial, and other defense mechanisms, as well as gain insight into their coping strategies and unique adjustments. These persons and their families have had to live with uncertainty. They may have received medical and psychological help, but they and their families, friends, and employers had to make their own way each day in dealing with the unfamiliar and unexpected as well as with the routine. This book may provide some guidance through the demanding terrain of this illness.

The frustrations of multiple sclerosis are real. The difficulty or impossibility of a long walk along a beach, the changing sensations that disturb one's rest at night, or the urgency to empty the bladder are real. No amount of words can cover that up. Nor should they. To deny the reality of that suffering is to deny you. It is part of your life. It is the stuff from which to forge your own truths about why and how you live. Regardless of your mobility, your strength, or your prognosis, that work is something no one can do for you.

But that does not mean to do it alone. It is our purpose in writing this book to show how the burden of multiple sclerosis—indeed, any catastrophe—can be borne more easily when there are others to share it with. And those who offer their resources, whether emotional, physical, financial, or spiritual, can also be enriched. We claim that the distinction between helper and helped may be a useful one, but it falls away in the face of our common human condition.

Many relationships become strained, even broken, from chronic illness. But with good information, sound advice, and examples of what others have accomplished, it is possible to keep going *and* growing. We hope this book will show you how.

LIVING WITH MULTIPLE SCLEROSIS

❖ 1 ❖

What Is Happening to Me?

THE INITIAL SIGNS of multiple sclerosis are strange and unpredictable. They may go as quickly as they come, leaving no clue as to their cause and whether they'll ever return. The trailing foot that never quite clears the next step or stumbles upon the crack in the sidewalk, pins and needles or excessive heat or cold or numbness in the hands, feet, arms, or legs—all are familiar first symptoms. A sensation of constant indigestion, never taking a comfortable deep breath, and a tightening around the trunk are other common early warning signals.

"I knew something was wrong when I was getting out of a hot bath one morning. My legs felt as if they had weights attached to them," reports Jonathan. He was unable to drive his car that day. Interestingly, Jonathan later discovered that one of the early tests for multiple sclerosis was to immerse people in warm water. If they became weaker as a result, it was considered a suggestive indication of possible M.S.

Sometimes the initial symptoms are more frightening. Double vision, blurring of vision, or even paralysis may occur, either temporarily—come and quickly go—or, on occasion, remain. "I was an illustrator," remembers Nicole, "and after a long day of drawing I was not surprised when my sight was a little blurry. One day, however, I had been at my board for barely twenty minutes when I had double vision. I rubbed my eyes, but it didn't go away. I figured maybe I had had too much coffee or perhaps I was getting a cold. I lay down for an hour, but couldn't stop opening my eyes to check my vision. It was still double.

"I called my boyfriend and he came over. By the time he arrived I had a headache, maybe as a result of my anxiety about my sight. Anyway, we figured my eye problems were probably a result of the headache and they disappeared after three or four hours.

"I thought nothing more of the incident until a month later when the double vision occurred again," Nicole goes on. "This time, however, it didn't go away the whole day, and since I couldn't work I went to an eye doctor. He couldn't find anything wrong with my vision beside my symptom, but he was concerned and alert enough to refer me to a neurologist. That started me down the road that eventually led to my M.S. diagnosis. The double vision improved, but other symptoms appeared that have left me unable to continue as a pen-and-ink illustrator. Fortunately I'm still able to use my graphic 'eye' and I now create computer-generated designs."

For the most part, M.S. approaches slowly, giving one no idea that something may be seriously wrong. Louise, a psychiatrist, was convinced that her urgency to urinate and slight abdominal discomfort were due to anxiety.

She attributed the weakness in her left leg to a "hysterical conversion reaction," or hysteria. Indeed, multiple sclerosis, with its "vague, multiple somatic symptoms," can raise some questions about psychological functioning. Fortunately, when Louise went to her physician, he refused to accept her self-diagnosis and referred her to a neurologist.

Because of the vagueness of the "multiple somatic symptoms," many people do not confide in their spouses, family, friends, or physician. They continue to think and, perhaps, hope that what they are experiencing is nothing more than tension or stress. Yet when symptoms do not clear up or they go away only to reappear at another time, one's unease increases. As Louise says, "I both wanted to know what was happening to me and I feared knowing it."

People are often reluctant to share their apprehension with loved ones because they want to protect them. They would like "it" all to just go away. And if that is not possible, most people want to take care of it by themselves and not be a bother to anyone. This is unfortunate, first, because it is not possible to manage the whole affair by oneself, and second, because it is not desirable to do so.

"When I first started getting strange 'cramping' and sensations at night and some urinary urgency, I was really concerned," Dick remembers. "But Linda was going through her own difficulties at work and I didn't want to add to her stress by bringing up my problems. I was afraid she might become sick herself if she had to worry about me. Besides, I wasn't so sure that what I was feeling was anything more than anxiety or a chronic flu.

"Sometimes, however, when she was telling me about her day, I'd become impatient with her for not noticing the apprehension I was feeling. I guess I needed some reassurance and mothering, and I expected Linda to see that that was what I wanted without having to tell her anything. I was in a lot of conflict between wanting to share with her and not wanting to burden her.

"Finally," Dick says, "I wet the bed one night. I felt so helpless and embarrassed and Linda was so surprised that I just had to tell her what I had been worrying about. Of course, as I should have known she would, she listened with real compassion; she didn't panic or get depressed. In fact, she was very firm with me about seeing a doctor to find out whether, indeed, there was anything wrong medically. It was interesting that once I was able to share my anxiety with her, I was bothered much less by her telling me about the pressures she was under. I guess once I felt my own vulnerability, I became more accepting of hers."

As we shall emphasize throughout this book, multiple sclerosis is a family affair and, in the most profound sense, like other chronic diseases, a family illness. The large web of family and social relations in which we all live is strained intensely when someone who is a part of it becomes sick. Sharing and communicating with each other is the way in which the web remains intact, and support, both practical and emotional, must be offered. Trust strengthens and silence weakens this network. The earlier that trust with intimates is established, the easier the journey with M.S. will be.

The decision to seek medical advice is a crucial time for a person with M.S. A bad experience with a physician may delay diagnosis and, even worse, leave one with a residue of anger and mistrust of "establishment" medicine and doctors that may never be healed. The fault for such outcomes lies with both the doctor and the patient.

Each has expectations of the other that are never met, and each has emotional defenses that remain unexamined.

"When I first went to a physician and told him about my symptoms," says Louise, "he referred me to a neurologist without the slightest hint of explanation. I told the neurologist that I thought my symptoms were signs of anxiety. What he did then, which I appreciate, is take the time to ask what I might be anxious about. After hearing me out, he said, 'Why must this be psychological?' I didn't feel so crazy after that."

Pleased that her symptoms were not psychosomatic, but anxious about their physical origin, Louise embarked on a medical journey peculiar to neurological illness in which one is less likely to be poked and prodded and asked about pain than one is to have wires attached and reflexes tested and to begin a slow process of ruling out one diagnosis after another. The uncertainty and length of time, often nearly two years, between the initial visit and the final pronouncement can be frustrating and maddening.

"I went into the hospital for the first time because I had weakness in my legs after swimming and a severe back pain that lasted all weekend," reports Pete, an accountant. "After two or three days of testing, the verdict was 'viral lesions of the spinal cord.' My neurologist said lots of people have them, but that it usually isn't discovered until an autopsy is done after death. 'Don't worry about it,' he said. 'No problem.' He said to call him if anything else occurs.

"During the next two years, the old symptoms continued and new ones appeared from time to time. 'Viral lesions of the spinal cord,' I told myself and my wife whenever I tried to understand what was happening.

Some symptoms I simply dismissed as anxiety. But then one hot summer day, while on vacation in the mountains, I tried to walk uphill, from the lake to my cabin. I just couldn't do it. My wife and kids, who were only eight and eleven at the time, had to help support and nearly drag me to the car. Once I cooled off my strength returned, so I just continued my vacation. Just another result of 'viral lesions of the spinal cord.'

"When I did go to my health plan the next week, the neurologist had me hospitalized and I once again underwent tests. This time the diagnosis was multiple sclerosis. I found out they had expected that all along, but no one told me! The doctors gave me their official reasons for not informing me of a suspected diagnosis. Nevertheless, I strongly feel I should have been told of any suspicions so I could have taken some measures to create more security for myself and my family.

"Like many self-employed individuals, I had no disability insurance and now, with a definite diagnosis, it would be nearly impossible or prohibitively expensive to obtain. My life insurance costs have also risen. And I might have taken a different approach to financial planning if my physicians had communicated their thoughts. Also, of course, I may have been diagnosed earlier if I didn't keep writing off my symptoms as due to 'viral lesions of the spinal cord.' I'm sure the doctors had good reasons for not being more open with me, but I think they ought to reconsider for the sake of others."

To seek medical advice can be a frightening experience. Louise's questions—What will the doctor do to me? What tests will I have? Do I need to be hospitalized? What will the diagnosis mean to my life? What kind of prognosis do I have for the future? Where or when should I get a second opinion? Why does it take so long to get answers?—were typical of individuals with multiple sclerosis in the late as well as the early stages of the disease. It is important for M.S. people and their families to understand the diagnostic procedures and process that neurologists use to confirm and follow the ongoing course of the disease.

Because M.S. symptoms are often vague and transient, people with M.S. and their families can easily discount them as purely psychological, or even hysterical, reactions while they await the physicians' diagnosis. Arm and leg numbness and sensations of pins and needles occur in many persons with psychosomatic disorders as well as in M.S. persons. Hyperventilation, which often accompanies these feelings, is also known to result from anxiety. As a result, the M.S. person can be wrongly labeled during the sometimes elongated time period it takes for the symptoms to be accurately diagnosed.

Each day then becomes a battle to balance precarious emotions and doubts as to what these symptoms really mean. These doubts consequently increase stress, which may in itself exacerbate the symptoms.

It was September, and Sybil's summer vacation had fast drawn to a close. In the first week of school, just when she most needed her strength for the onslaught of thirty new second graders, her legs began to feel strange again. They became numb and heavy. "It became difficult for me to even drag them up the stairs to arrive at my second-floor classroom," she admitted to her friend, Sue, who taught next door.

As she rushed around her classroom, feelings of pins and needles began again in both legs. Sybil felt as if both legs had fallen asleep and they were difficult to arouse. Finally the children had recess, and Sybil could relax for a few minutes. When the children returned to the classroom, however, she found herself involuntarily inhaling and exhaling at a rapid pace. "I'm hyperventilating," she admitted to Sue in awe. "Was I so tense about my legs that my anxiety took over?"

At Sue's suggestion, both women went to the principal's office. Sybil thought it was only fair to alert Mr. Spencer to her dilemma. This was only the first week of school. She didn't know if she could continue through the entire year. Just this thought made her so tense that she found herself breathless as she approached his office.

This kind, elderly gentleman listened carefully to Sybil's explanation of her problem. Though he respected her professional abilities, he found himself wondering about this attractive, forty-year-old woman who had never married. Was this tension reflective of her social anxieties, and not her physical condition at all? He found himself more doubtful of her symptoms as the interview continued, and finally, gently yet forcefully, he inquired, "Sybil, instead of the internist who you have been seeing about these problems, have you considered a psychiatrist?"

Sybil was crushed but not surprised. His response validated her own self-doubts. The medical tests she had had that summer had all been negative. Was Mr. Spencer right? Did her symptoms have a psychological basis? In response, Sybil became tearful and frustrated at her lack of professionalism.

After a few more months Sybil's internist finally sent her for a neurological consultation. This specialist then began a process of evaluating her, and reached the diagnosis of multiple sclerosis.

* * *

Most commonly, multiple sclerosis is diagnosed and managed by neurologists; these are physicians specially trained in physical and chemical disorders of the brain, spinal cord, and other nervous tissue. As a specialist, the neurologist will take a very complete medical history of all current symptoms and related or past health problems. The doctor wants to know when and under what circumstances symptoms appear. Is there a family history of any neurological disease, including M.S.? Have there been intermittent symptoms in the past that were overlooked? The doctor needs to know if you've experienced any functional changes in your ability to carry out daily activities. What gives you the most difficulty at home or work are helpful pieces in the solving of the puzzle that leads to a diagnosis. Casting doubt and critically questioning a previous diagnosis of M.S. is the hallmark of a good and objective physician. The thinking doctor knows multiple sclerosis may be erroneously diagnosed or overlooked by other M.D.s.

After the medical history comes physical and neurological examinations. The doctor is particularly interested in looking into your eyes with a small ophthalmoscope light to see if the optic nerve is pale, causing a blur or blind spot in your vision. He looks for diplopia (double vision), a weakness in eye movements, and jiggling of the eyes called nystagmus. He also listens to the clarity of speech for any thickness or slurring. Reflexes are evaluated with a reflex hammer. Muscle strength is checked in arms and legs, each muscle being tested individually. The legs are looked at for stiffness and spasticity. Sensation is tested by a light touch, a gentle pinprick, a positional movement of your toe up and down, and with soft vibrations from a tuning fork. The smoothness of coordination is seen in how you reach a finger from your nose to the doctor's finger and how you slide the heel of one foot down the shin of the opposite leg. Your ability to walk and maintain balance is examined.

The purpose of this exam, and similar ones that will continue throughout the course of the illness, is to determine if there has been more than one attack in time and if more than one area of the nervous system has been affected in space. At least two events in time and space in the central nervous system are needed as minimal criteria to even suspect M.S. in most cases. This fact helps to understand why the diagnosis may take months, or even years, to confirm. Until there are multiple attacks in space and time, affecting brain, spinal cord, or optic nerves, the diagnosis remains in doubt.

But even this information is usually not sufficient to make a firm diagnosis. To be sure that a different condition is not masquerading as M.S. and to avoid telling someone he or she has M.S. when only "sound alike" symptoms are present, certain tests may be necessary on an outpatient basis or in the hospital. A lumbar puncture (spinal tap) is done to examine spinal fluid. It is usually performed under local anesthetic and involves minimal discomfort.

In the laboratory, the fluid is examined for an increased number of cells, especially lymphocytes, which are part of the immune system that makes antibodies, against your own myelin. Chemical analyses are conducted for abnormal quantities of certain proteins known as myelin basic protein, immunoglobulins, or oligoclonal bands. These different proteins may be more prevalent with chronic progressive M.S. or during an attack of acute M.S.

Multiple lesions may be confirmed in most M.S. patients with harmless, noninvasive studies, which may include electroencephalogram (EEG, or so-called brain waves) and evoked responses. These tests tell how fast or slow electrical activity occurs in the nervous system. The evoked responses may be delayed between one point and another in the visual, brain stem, and spinal areas. A tiny electrical signal evokes an electrical response on a screen.

A CAT scan picture of the brain taken after contrast dye has been injected intravenously may show multiple areas that "light up," distinguishing M.S. from other conditions that are also "multiple," like strokes or tumors. Blood tests are drawn to rule out conditions that might slow you down, like an underactive thyroid or anemia.

The object is to rule out alternative diagnostic possibilities and to rule in multiple sclerosis only if it is possible, probable, or definite by medical criteria. In this way, errors in diagnosis are usually avoided. As you may surmise by now, the multiple findings may not all be present when you first see your doctor or have your first test. Don't let delays due to exactness discourage you. It may not be possible to establish a sure diagnosis until a second attack occurs, which may not happen for months or years.

Once a diagnosis is made the physician can talk about treatment options and alternatives, including whether or not treatment needs to begin immediately. The many choices of treatment will be explained. What cannot be treated will also be explained. What you should worry about and what you should not worry about may be clarified. The chance of a spontaneous remission with all signs and symptoms disappearing for a while is always possible. Remissions are common occurrences. And when symptoms reappear, a different treatment approach may be recommended.

While the doctor is busy examining and sifting the data, he may not be able to give immediate answers or explanations. He is not being evasive or aloof; he is just trying to be an objective professional. When all the information is in, he will be able to sit down and explain what it all means to you and your family. That is the time to ask all your questions. Just keep in mind that some of them may not be answerable. A world of patience and tolerance on your part is needed so the careful and lengthy process gets done properly.

It is very important for you and your doctor to work out a relationship based on confidence, competency, and trust. The need for such an exchange, in fact, rests more upon the person with multiple sclerosis than it does upon the professional caregiver. It is your responsibility to find a physician with whom you can feel comfortable in that kind of close relationship. If your existing doctor meets your needs, fine. If not, then be a smart consumer and search for someone who does.

It is best if the neurologist is familiar with multiple sclerosis and up-to-date with the latest information and treatments. Your local chapter of the National Multiple Sclerosis Society (see Appendix) should be able to provide you with the names of such physicians.

The relief that a diagnosis may bring is, of course, transcended by the initial reaction to the naming of the illness. Confusion, panic, despair, and anger are all understandable reactions. But perhaps the most common reaction is what psychologists call denial. Denial is a psychological defense mechanism that people employ to avoid acknowledging a painful event. It is a method people use to adapt to events that are too terrible to accept all at once.

"When my M.S. was finally diagnosed," reports Louise, "I just said to myself, 'Okay, that's it. Fine, let's just get on with living. A minor annoyance, nothing else.' With my psychological toughness, I felt I could cope with anything that small. If I didn't have that certainty, I probably would have become quite withdrawn, perhaps turned to my books searching for an answer to 'why me?'

"In looking back, I can see that my denial of the seriousness of my illness gave me the time and energy to make a substantial number of changes in my life. I took a sabbatical from work, I told myself, to do research. In fact, it gave me the time I needed to confront more realistically my M.S."

Sometimes short-term denial is a way station to dealing with a crisis and, as in Louise's case, can be beneficial. Long-term denial, however, makes useful action more difficult. Instead of making a problem disappear, denial simply makes it worse. Joe, for example, is a man proud of his masculine approach to life. For him, sickness was a sign of weakness. When he began to stumble, he preferred to let his neighbors think he was drunk rather than visit a doctor. Once he saw a physician and received a diagnosis of multiple sclerosis, *he continued to tell people that his falls were due to alcohol* to avoid admitting that he was sick.

In Joe's case, sickness conflicted with an ideal of masculine invulnerability that accepted excessive drinking as a legitimate behavior. Only when Joe found a journal his adolescent daughter kept, in which she expressed her anguish about how the neighbors viewed her "alcoholic" father, did he confront his denial. Joe was never able to understand his daughter's disappointment in his actions until he saw her journal. Though he had listened to her in the past, he had never before listened with his heart. He felt she was being a "typical teen," overcritical of actions that were none of her concern. Physical prowess had always been essential to Joe's concept of his own adequacy. He grew up as a macho type of athletic youngster. His strength was a source of pride for his parents. Though his grades were never terrific, his father took great pleasure in watching him play center on the local high school football team. "I earned three letters in high school," he would boast to old friends, "and I certainly think I made the difference in many championship teams."

After high school, Joe elected to remain in the same community and drive a truck. He soon owned several trucks of his own, and established a moving company. His strength with even the heaviest furniture was well known. He would assure new customers that "this is the only moving company that would not fold if all employees did not show up for work. I could take care of all jobs single-handedly." His burly form and ready laugh were always visible in town. Joe greatly exceeded his modest vocational aspirations as his moving business became more and more successful.

Joe was diagnosed with multiple sclerosis several years ago, when both of his daughters were in elementary school. After the first attack he went into remission, and so his denial phase was extended and unquestioned. The pain of adjusting to a chronic disease, especially one that could change his entire physical presentation, was too much to bear. Several years later, Joe experienced two exacerbations in the same year. His legs were affected; not only was he now limited in his gait, but he was unable to work in his usual capacity. He continued to refuse to admit to physical weakness, and though confronted by this reality for several months in a row, he forbade his wife and daughters from sharing the truth with anyone else. He was far more comfortable blaming his behavior on the tensions of business, which led him to alcohol "for relaxation." His identification of illness with weakness and his patterns of psychological cover-up were so strong that it took a long period of counseling before he would acknowledge his disease and accept multiple sclerosis as a legitimate aspect of himself.

Many people with multiple sclerosis continue to behave in ways that are comfortable and reassuring to themselves, yet refuse to face the painful facts of their illness, and thus deprive themselves of having their real needs met. Bert is another man whose denial continued to be maladaptive. Being sick, from Bert's point of view, meant that "my life 'was not working,' that I wasn't 'on the right track.' As a result, I was ashamed that I had become sick and that kept me from acknowledging to myself or the people close to me what had happened. I thought if I just corrected my life-style I'd be okay. When the M.S. didn't go away, I was really knocked for a loop and I was afraid and ashamed to tell my friends about it. I thought they'd reject me as someone who 'couldn't get it together.' "

Bert's denial kept him from getting the physical and emotional support that would have been helpful to him in the early stages of his illness. Whereas Joe identified illness with weakness, Bert identified it with wrongness. His idea of physical health was strongly equated with moral goodness. He maintained a primitive concept in which "gods" or "life" punished people with misfortunes for poor psychological attitudes. Failure to get what he wanted in life, whether in relationships, finances, or fitness, indicated spiritual weakness. Bert had a grandiose notion of his ability to manipulate reality to conform to his desires.

The belief that one's attitude and emotions can affect

one's physical health and either cause or cure disease is very popular in our culture. It also has the potential to be a very dangerous idea. For example, not only may people blame themselves for their illness, as Bert did, but they may undergo a great deal of unnecessary suffering and, in some cases, fail to obtain adequate medical care.

Patricia was diagnosed with multiple sclerosis while she was involved with a "new age" group that emphasized the power of positive thinking. "My chief symptom was weakness in my legs. The leader of my group told me that my illness was the result of my failure to take a 'stand for myself' in my life. He said as long as I continued to live my life in my 'old' way, my illness would remain. Since I already believed that I was totally responsible for my health, I agreed with him. I changed my life-style; I started using megavitamins and macrobiotic foods. Of course, my M.S. didn't change as a result, so I just switched to other techniques—hypnosis, meditation, more personal growth courses—but nothing did the trick. I even fasted. My physical health apart from the M.S. began to deteriorate.

"Meanwhile, my family and closest friends were concerned that I was spending too much money and time running from one thing to another. I got angry at them for raising their objections. I was convinced that I was just not trying hard enough and my self-esteem plummeted.

"Fortunately," says Patricia, "I agreed to go to a therapist who helped me make contact with the M.S. Society. He also found out quite a bit about M.S. I learned that neither my personality nor my life-style caused my M.S., nor could they cure it. I understood that I could improve my overall physical fitness and adopt a mental attitude that could help me function as well as possible within the physical limits imposed by my disease. I stopped blaming myself and started dealing with what I had. My denial was expressed through my hoping to find some kind of 'magic cure' or 'white knight' healer. When I started talking to people outside my groups I got some good advice and lots of support."

Knowing whom, when, and what to tell about one's condition is often difficult. When Jonathan was first diagnosed, he told most people that his shaky gait and occasional stumbles were due to "nerve damage." He was not yet comfortable with the diagnosis and avoided any further discussion by referring to a vague condition. It also referred to something stable rather than progressive and injury-related rather than disease. Obviously, Jonathan himself felt much more at ease thinking of his illness that way.

After every explanation of nerve damage, Jonathan's wife would ask him why he used that term, and he would rationalize by telling her how much more comfortable other people were when he described his difficulties that way. Jonathan's wife had moved beyond the state of denial and wanted him to face up to the reality of his disease. As we shall discuss in Chapter 2, one partner is very often ahead of the other in moving through the stages of adaptation to multiple sclerosis and other chronic diseases.

Jonathan soon began to abandon his nerve-damage defense, and started telling almost everyone he met that he had M.S. He would describe the disease, the diagnostic process, theories of causation and cure, and his own prognosis. Occasionally, his wife or one of his listeners would remark upon the incongruent yet pleasant smile that seemed to accompany his brief discourse.

When they heard his diagnosis, both family and

friends were distraught and extended support in all kinds of ways ranging from giving him the name of acupuncturists and chiropractors to holding prayer circles or offering financial aid. Jonathan felt very uncomfortable with all these gestures. People seemed to take his illness more seriously than he did, and his facade of unconcern began to crack. The euphoria with which he reported his illness masked his anxiety.

Although it was helpful for Jonathan to view his illness more seriously, "the distress of my family and friends seemed out of proportion to my actual medical situation. I was embarrassed by the offers of help, and types of healing I could not agree with, from people I barely knew. My private difficulties had become a public event. I wished I had been more discriminating in whom I confided."

The euphoric feeling that often accompanies and is a sign of denial is typical. It is as if a person with pneumonia goes hatless on windy days to demonstrate his confidence in his recovery. Shortly after diagnosis, people may say or do things that seem foolish from a more objective stance. Concerned others may also feel taken in by the ill person, who intimately describes details one moment but rarely reveals anything after that.

"Indeed," says Jonathan, "it was not unusual for me to avoid my listeners after that. I had a sense of having gone too far, as if I had been on a bender and didn't want to see anyone who might have noticed." It is wise to limit your confidences to a few people with whom you are sure to share a few months or years down the road. The reason many people describe thoughts of "healing" you is often the result of their own anxiety concerning your well-being and future. A visible disability or illness gives other people the opportunity to determine how much they want to know. For many people with M.S., others are unaware of the illness unless they are specifically told.

It is important to let the people close to you know how you are doing. Because M.S. is such an unpredictable and confusing disease, your friends and family can't know what to expect or how to respond unless you tell them. Rosalyn was married for three years when she was diagnosed with multiple sclerosis. Her husband, Steven, was quite supportive and compassionate and remained deeply committed to their marriage. But Rosalyn had never felt comfortable with her in-laws.

"I didn't want to tell them," she explains, "because I was afraid they would use the information against Steven and me. They never hid their belief that he had not picked the right girl when we chose to marry. They would subtly encourage a separation, especially because they had not yet had grandchildren."

Rosalyn's in-laws regularly served buffet meals on special occasions. Although they noticed the difficulty Rosalyn had standing in line and manipulating her silverware and plate, they attributed the symptoms to "nerves" and "laziness." They never asked what was wrong, nor did they alter their customary service. Steven did not tell them out of respect for Rosalyn's wishes. Yet she became increasingly resentful of their lack of sensitivity.

"One day Steven confronted me about the game I was playing with his parents," Rosalyn comments. "He said I expected them to be mind readers and got angry with them when they were not. He was right. He knew about my fear of their turning him away from me. He said he was totally committed to our marriage. We decided to tell them together.

"I was really nervous the day I sat in their living room. Steven began the conversation by telling them of how deeply we loved each other and acknowledging their hesitancy in supporting our relationship. He said that whatever they thought was their business, but how they acted toward me was his. Then I told them about the M.S. I told them as much as I knew, and that it was unlikely to interfere with my ability to have children. Simply the thought that we were planning children seemed to relax them, and they began to ask questions.

"I can't say our relationship warmed up overnight," Rosalyn continues, "but they did seem to make efforts to be more helpful. The next meal at their house was a sit-down dinner, and I thanked Steven's mother for thinking about me. In retrospect, I wished I had told them earlier and let the chips fall where they may."

Jonathan spoke too freely and Rosalyn was not forthcoming enough. As each became more able to share with the important people in their lives and became psychologically adjusted to their chronic illness, they each became more connected and relaxed with family and friends.

Some people's problems with communicating about their illness are complicated by their being single. Amy's story reveals a few of these issues: "I'm a dancer and my initial symptoms were fatigue and loss of strength and coordination in my right leg. The symptoms had persisted for over a year so, of course, I suspected that it was not a temporary disability caused by overwork. But to hear the confirmation and the labeling . . . multiple sclerosis . . . my lifelong dream, my art, my career were shattered.

"I went home and told my fiancé. He said very little. He had become irritated lately by my complaints. I thought he'd be relieved to know that I was not some hypochondriac but the possessor of a real disease. The next day he left. He was angry with me. He said I had no right to expect him to sacrifice his whole life for me." The harsh anger of Amy's fiancé indicated that he was denying his anxiety about illness and disability and projecting the reason for his discomfort onto Amy.

Confused and hurt by her fiancé's reaction, Amy got tough. She made it a policy to tell the men she met that she had multiple sclerosis at the very beginning of their relationships, despite the fact that her illness did not interfere with her social life. She challenged men to be as "strong" as she was in accepting her disability and dismissed them as weak when they withdrew.

Only with counseling did Amy see that she was not as accepting of her disease as she thought, but was very angry, fearful, and sad about it. The feelings she denied were projected onto her male friends just as her fiancé had cast his emotional conflicts upon her. She actually felt quite unacceptable as a "handicapped" person, and pushed potential friends away to avoid burdening them with her needs. Amy had to come to terms with her M.S. and its blow to her self-image as a graceful and competent person.

Amy was unnecessarily demanding when she forced people to relate to her on the basis of her illness before they had learned about each other as people. What she interpreted as men's withdrawal because of her disease could just as easily been interpreted as their moving away from her forced and premature need for intimacy.

Once Amy let people get to know her before disclosing her multiple sclerosis, her social life went more smoothly. She no longer classified men simply as "weak" or "strong," but began to appreciate both individual weaknesses and strengths. Building on a foundation of trust, she and the men she became involved with could discuss mutual responses to her illness more easily.

People tend to deny their own anxiety about illness and disability. They have powerful and complex thoughts and feelings about those whose misfortunes bring to mind the possibility of being subject to a similar fate. When such strong emotion is also associated with dating and sexuality, the special problems of developing a social life with a physical hardship become clear. We strongly suggest that a single person seek a counselor who is aware of these special problems that are, we think, unique. Therapists whose experience and training does not include work with the ill or physically challenged is usually missing a dimension that a single person with multiple sclerosis needs.

Other people's responses, no matter how well meaning, can carry negative messages. People whose only knowledge of M.S. is having known or seen someone with a very advanced case imagine that all people become wheelchair bound and extremely disabled. They are not aware of all the people with invisible, mild, or moderate M.S. They are alarmist in their expectations and ought to be immediately and straightforwardly corrected, lest they contribute to unnecessary fear, and even panic.

Doug remembers, "When I told my parents of my M.S. diagnosis, my mother went into what I can only describe as shock. They wondered what would become of my wife and my children without a father, that I was too young, that they felt the worse curse was to outlive a child. I couldn't understand their reactions.

"I called my sister that first evening to tell her my diagnosis and I also spoke to her of the way my parents took the news. She said that they had already called her in an absolute panic and had made her very fearful as well. I asked her from where they could have gotten their notion of M.S. She remembered that she had once been at a family affair where there had been a relative in a wheelchair. She thought she had been told the person had multiple sclerosis or something like that, which meant nothing to her at the time.

"I followed up with a phone call to my parents," says Doug, "and asked if they had ever known anyone with M.S. They said there had been a son of a cousin who had it, but he had died some years before. They thought he had moved from being an active fellow to a wheelchair rather quickly and had died within a very few years of his diagnosis. That was not only what they feared, but what they *expected* to happen to me. Their model for my M.S. was a worse-case scenario they had seen many years before.

"I reassured them that our cousin had been unusually unfortunate, and that my outcome was likely to be much better, based on my conversations with my physician. I realized that just as I had needed to find out about M.S., they had the same need as well. I needed to correct their ideas before they spread misinformation and panic throughout the family. I went over that very night and asked them what they knew about M.S. I corrected anything I knew to be wrong and told them I'd get the information about anything I didn't know.

"I think my lack of fear and willingness to talk with them about their concerns reduced their anxiety considerably. In fact," Doug concludes, "they became experts of their own sort on M.S., joined the Society, learned whatever they could, and became local fundraisers. They used my M.S. as a way of becoming of some service to others."

Marshall recalls Seth, a fellow worker at a travel

agency. Seth was a good travel agent, meticulous with figures, knowledgeable about the computer, and an experienced traveler himself—in short, in possession of most traits necessary to be efficient and productive in the travel agent business. One day Seth complained about double vision and some mild eyestrain. Further, he complained about fatigue from sitting, concentrating, working, etc. After several days with the same symptoms, Seth finally decided to pay a visit to his family doctor, who sent him to a neurologist. Seth was diagnosed with M.S. of the chronic-progressive type. Within six months Seth was working only part-time, and he had to rest several hours each day to maintain even these reduced hours. He was in a wheelchair within the first year, and by the second year, Seth was totally unable to continue working. Whenever Marshall heard someone refer to M.S., he thought of Seth.

Three years after this episode, Marshall's wife, Joyce, was diagnosed with this same disease. Her symptoms were different from Seth's, the progression was slower, and her ability to maintain her work schedule remained intact; nonetheless, whenever Joyce wanted to speak about her illness, her fatigue, or frustration with a chronic disease, Marshall could only recall Seth. As a result, he became angry. Joyce could not understand the extent of her husband's anger. She always considered Marshall to be a patient and understanding man. Yet he continued to visualize Seth and his downward progression with a severe case of M.S. whenever his wife needed help in coping with her symptoms.

In addition to her own anger in adjusting to M.S., Joyce had to deal with her husband's angry outbursts. She naturally assumed that his temper was addressed solely at her. She would become silent and more distant from him at these times. It took many months and much supportive therapy from professionals who were knowledgeable about the adjustment process of a chronic disease for Joyce and Marshall to understand differently. "I finally realized that Marshall was not angry with me at all," Joyce admitted to her therapist, "but with the negative memories of Seth that M.S. symptoms invoked in him. He was so fearful that I would progress along the same course Seth did."

In fact, Marshall was fearful and anxious about multiple sclerosis. He felt helpless in being unable to help his wife and alter what he had wrongly assumed was a disastrous and inevitable course.

Some people recommend cures—diets, exercises, philosophies, healers, medicine—that have worked for them or people they have known or heard about. Although it is normal and sensible to want to seek all possible remedies, it is expensive, time consuming, and almost invariably fruitless.

In adjusting to M.S., many people go through a "bargaining" stage where they unrealistically wish for a miracle cure to alter the diagnosis. Marcia was in just this stage as she read a well-written advertisement in a Florida newspaper. It described a specially processed type of snake venom that was almost "guaranteed" to cure diseases. She scanned the list of illnesses that would promptly disappear with treatment; M.S. was among them. The cost of the treatment was $350 in addition to transportation and motel charges.

Marcia was a clerk in a local clothing store. She made just enough money each month to buy food, pay rent, and make car payments. Because Marcia was conscientious, she never overbought or fell behind in her responsibilities.

This "treatment trip," as she lovingly began to call it, would put her finances in arrears for the next six months;

she would have to use her car payment money to pay for her plane fare and the treatment she desperately desired. After fantasizing for a few days, Marcia decided that "it is finally time to do something positive for myself," as she explained to her mother, who was shocked at her daughter's impractical rashness. "It can't hurt and will probably help," Marcia explained with joy.

Marcia was vulnerable and gullible. This well-written ad that remained unaccompanied by medical documentation had convinced her to spend hundreds of dollars that she did not have in order to find a medical cure for her disease. She found none.

Before spending money and energy chasing down other people's suggestions, contact the local chapter of the Multiple Sclerosis Society and ask them what their research indicates about your potential cure.

That there is no medical cure to M.S. is very frustrating. There may be mistrust of the medical establishment, which developed out of the difficult prediagnostic period, but that is no excuse for frantically and compulsively tracking down every cure that anybody has ever heard of. That is lunacy.

It is important to screen the useful from the unnecessary information, the positive from the despairing suggestions. As the veil of denial begins to lift, it becomes easier to determine what is plausible. One begins to look at the course of one's illness with a more realistic perspective, and getting lost in the trap of false hope is less likely. There is less anxiety about whether one's multiple sclerosis will disappear forever or whether one is inevitably doomed to immobility and blindness. Instead, there is acceptance of the unknowable and unexpected nature of M.S. and a determination to live a good, compassionate, and useful life. Such a life need not be bound by physical constraints.

❖ 2 ❖

What Is Happening to You?

THE SERIOUS ILLNESS of a spouse or other loved one is one of the most highly stressful events that a person can undergo. Couples must cope with many practical concerns—medical care, financial resources, potential career or job shifts are a few. They must also face, as a couple and as individuals, the highly complex and emotional dynamics that swirl around and inside us at times of crisis. Innumerable demands are made on our time and energy, and many solutions to particular problems give rise to new difficulties that must also be met. Sadness, guilt, anger, despair, and confusion are all typical feelings associated with the losses that chronic illness and abrupt change bring. Hopefulness, love, compassion, and support are also emotions that are richly present when life's unwelcome certainties (for pain, suffering, aging, and loss are assured) intrude into our lives.

The illness of a partner is filled with paradoxes. "It wasn't me who was sick," points out Mark, "but I experienced my wife's discomfort as my own. Liz was ill, yet I seemed more concerned than she. In some ways I had to make even more changes in my life-style than did my ill companion. I had to be prepared if her functioning deteriorated. Although the diagnosis was my loved one's rather than my own, all but the actual symptoms became part of my life. And when the stress of the whole business began to wear away at me, I even developed an assortment of physical symptoms. We were obliged to have joint custody of Liz's illness.

"Liz was already at home taking care of the children as a homemaker. There's no question that with her M.S. her job was more difficult and she needed to rest more often. So I had to modify my work schedule to be more available during the week and on weekends to help out with the kids. Since Liz couldn't drive because of the effect M.S. had on her vision, I had to do a lot more dropping off and picking up. Although the neighbors were quite helpful, I had to fill in on field trips, ball games, and school activities.

"I also had to help out more with the cleaning," Mark continues. "We had fairly defined roles until then, so although my head told me what I should do, it took some time for me to get used to doing some of what I suppose I should have been doing all along, even if Liz had not become sick."

"I have to give Mark a lot of credit," offers Liz. "We're a pretty traditional couple and we were both satisfied with how we had split our roles up. But the M.S. just made it impossible for us to continue as before. I know Mark was angry that he had to pitch in with more of the childcare and housework than he was used to. He was also anxious that his career might suffer if he had to spend more time with us.

"I love him and I was willing to put up with some of the irritation and difficulties he was going through, but there came a point when I had to confront him. I didn't choose to be sick. I wasn't pushing him to be a more at-home dad. It just had to be done. We became tense with each other for a while. But I must admit, he came around a lot quicker than I expected. He got rid of his attitude of self-pity and blaming and settled down to do what needed to be done."

It is especially important for the people on the outside—family, friends, colleagues—to recognize the shared impact of M.S. and other chronic illnesses upon both members of a couple. It is even more necessary, of course, for couples themselves to understand how the presence of an illness brings with it responsibility and opportunity for both mourning tattered dreams and weaving new hopes for the unknown future.

"When John told me the neurologist's diagnosis of M.S.," Sherry recounts, "we were totally unprepared. I knew so little about the disease; I was shocked and frightened for John, for our children, for myself. The only images I had were of very disabled, wheelchair-bound people, and that's where I kept seeing John. I felt so sad for him.

"Something curious gradually started to happen," notes Sherry. "I didn't want to believe it was true, that it was some bad dream. But at the same time, another part of my mind and heart were saying that it was true, that I had to be strong to take care of my husband, to help bring him to health.

"John kept telling me not to worry, that it wasn't so bad, his case was mild, and so on. He kept minimizing any concerns or feelings I had. He seemed ready to go on with his life, but I wasn't. As much as I feared knowing, I wanted to learn as much as I could about M.S., and it seemed as if he couldn't be bothered. When I did press him to find out more or talk to me about his feelings, he got irritated, accused me of being hysterical, and pulled away. I was terribly hurt and angry when he did this; he was denying both of us the support we needed to share."

Both John and Sherry's reactions are typical. John is demonstrating the euphoria and denial stage that was described in Chapter 1. The doctor had told him the facts, and since there was nothing to be done about it, John wasn't going to waste any energy worrying about multiple sclerosis. He'd act as if his limp was nothing more than a pulled muscle or bad sprain.

Because John refused to acknowledge the anxiety he felt about his health and his future, Sherry's questions touched the exposed nerve of his insecurity and fear. His irritation was the reflexive response of a person whose image of himself as healthy and in control was under attack. Although Sherry interpreted John's anger as directed at her, it was actually directed at the images of illness and loss of control that threatened his self-regard.

"Sometimes, when John turned away from me," Sherry continues, "I tried to get close again, begging him to talk with me. It seemed like the closer I tried to get the more he withdrew. After a while, I wouldn't say anything at all about the M.S. Interestingly, I noticed we were arguing more about other things—small, petty things that would have gone unnoticed before."

John sought emotional distance when he felt tension within himself or between himself and Sherry. When Sherry was anxious, on the other hand, she felt more comfortable closing the distance between herself and another. The dysfunctional pattern of interaction that

John and Sherry set up is obvious. His attempts to withdraw provoked her pursuit, which resulted in his moving even further away. Unfortunately, neither John nor Sherry were aware that their well-meaning individual solutions to their emotional distress created problems for them as a couple.

The ongoing touchiness and arguments about previously trivial matters were an active residue of the jumble of guilt, anger, sadness, and frustration they each felt but were unable to express and acknowledge to each other. If John had been more willing to confront and confide his concerns to Sherry, and if Sherry more easily realized that much of her pushing of John to open up was her own struggle to deal with her conflicting feelings toward John and his M.S., their interactions would have been more successful.

One area that is of particular difficulty for spouses of those with multiple sclerosis is coping with some of the more common symptoms. Occasional incontinence, stumbling, or dropping of silverware are no more than minor annoyances compared to the potential gravity of M.S., but they may be major sources of embarrassment.

"I felt angry at John for his accidents," says Sherry, "and I thought he could have done more to prevent them. 'Why didn't you make sure you used the rest room before we left? Why did you forget your cane? Why don't you remember to take a nap?' were all questions I'd ask in my frustration. Of course, he was feeling terrible as it was, and I'd feel guilty and ashamed for getting angry with him."

There is a valuable message in Sherry's questions to John. His lack of precaution was a result of his denial of his M.S. and its symptoms. Although it often occurred to him to take the preventative steps suggested by Sherry, he refused because it would mean "giving in" to his illness. Latent hostility, however, emerges at times in the tone of Sherry's questioning. The hostility is an expression of the conflict Sherry experienced when her image of herself as a caring wife and person was contradicted by the anger and embarrassment she felt at John's actions. The resentment she felt at being deprived of a healthy husband and easy future is also an understandable, yet often suppressed, source of disaffection.

The pictures we have of ourselves in our roles as spouses, companions, and lovers are constantly being challenged by the ever-present and ever-changing demands of living with chronic illness. When we perceive ourselves as not living up to our self-described role obligations we feel guilty; we feel anger toward those who we believe either fail to recognize our roles or whose behavior "forces" us to act in ways that are incongruent with our self-expectations.

Jay and Diane were together as college students, probably as much due to need as for enjoyment. He was organized, efficient, and compulsive about his studies. Each weekend evening, while his roommates were planning their outings, he was on his way to the library. At first they invited him to go along, but after continual refusals, they stopped. By January, everyone in the apartment knew that Jay was headed to the library; his friends had distinctly separate plans.

One snowy evening he looked up as he heard a book fall at the same time a woman muttered, "Damn, I'm sorry. I came all this way without a notebook and pen. Can I borrow some of that clean, lined paper?" Jay had to laugh at the sight of Diane, armed with too much equipment in too little order. As if she could read his expression, she added, "Can you believe that I lugged all this stuff through the snow and still can't find what I need?" Then, instead of worrying about it, as he would, she began to laugh. "I joined her, and had a good belly laugh for the first time in months," he recalls.

That was the beginning of a firm, complementary relationship. Diane was gregarious, fun, carefree, and totally spontaneous. Her grades, however, reflected this style. When a friend entered her room at any hour, despite any plans she may have had to study, that friend became the priority. As a result, she knew half the campus after just a few months into her freshman year. "I was always amazed at how many people spoke to her each day," Jay recalls. "I felt so good walking beside her. People actually noticed me for the first time, out of class."

Diane's grades were always precarious. She needed someone to organize her work, help her plan her time, and quiz her on material; she had to talk out her classwork in order for it to make sense. "We soon became inseparable," Diane agrees. "He seemed to need my socialization skills as much as I needed him to organize me. I continually learned from him.

"Our engagement did not surprise any of our friends. We planned to marry the week after graduation. It seemed perfect. How could we get along without each other? We seemed only half-people when we weren't together." Thus Diane aptly summed up the complementary, somewhat dependent approach to life that she and Jay had developed in three and a half years of togetherness.

Jay picks up the story at this point. "You see, I planned to continue helping Diane throughout our lives. We used to laugh a lot in those days as we planned to move into a neighborhood and send her right out to ring doorbells in order to make friends for us. I would stay home, we agreed, to unpack and make our home livable. We both knew that if she put things away we'd never find them again."

As things happened, Diane and Jay did not marry as they had planned. Two weeks before their wedding, Jay fell—he seemed to trip over his own foot—and broke his leg. While he was in the hospital, with time to think about himself, he admitted to Diane that he had been having a hard time focusing his eyes. Sometimes the printed page looked blurry, and on occasion he even had double vision. "I was sure he needed glasses," Diane responds at this point in the story. "He always studied too hard. Eyestrain was my explanation."

Jay did not overtly disagree with his fiancée. But for several weeks he had suspected that something more complex medically was going on with him. "I seemed clumsier than usual, always tripping over scatter rugs in the apartment and other foolish things like that. I was scared to go to the doctor," he admitted.

After a while Diane began to worry, too. "The diagnosis of M.S. took so long," she complains. Finally, after several months of uncertainty and continual symptoms, the neurologist from the hospital summoned Jay and Diane together to hear the story. "He was frank, though gentle with us," she recalls. "He explained that, at this point, it was difficult to predict what type of M.S. Jay had—not all types have poor prognoses. But he was clear about certain things that we would have to adjust to," she adds. Jay's doctor attempted to prepare them for the predisposition to fatigue that often accompanies the disease. "He also talked about the double vision and accompanying eye problems that can make it difficult to read during an attack. By the time he suggested that Jay use a cane so he wouldn't trip as often, I couldn't listen anymore," Diane admits. "I kept wondering what would happen to me. I had grown to rely on Jay to help me. Did all this mean he would have to rely on me?"

Diane never felt she was self-sufficient, nor had she matured to achieve competency in anything. She wrongly believed that she had someone with her who could always take over. "I felt so vulnerable. I was too worried about myself to even empathize with Jay," she recalls.

Diane and Jay began to argue in earnest for the first time. "The differences between us that had before seemed so cute and funny were now scary," Jay admits. "How could I let her take over when I was sick?" Then Jay began to feel guilty both about his negative, angry feelings toward Diane as well as his abandonment of her care. "I always promised to take care of her," he explains, "and now, because of this unexpected disease, I wasn't able to keep all my promises."

Instead of aiming to develop into mutually supportive independent persons, Jay had continued where Diane's parents had left off. He had encouraged her dependency on him. At the time it flattered his ego, but in making him feel good, she was developing a type of learned helplessness, unable to function as a mature adult. Now that he was sick and required a mate who was an adult, he became increasingly more critical and dissatisfied with her childish role. Though Jay had assisted in stereotyping Diane, he was no longer satisfied to marry this type of personality. He needed a more self-sufficient wife who would be able to share responsibilities with him.

The couple entered into therapy, and after several visits with a therapist, they both understood that their marriage would not be of benefit for either of them at this time. Diane had developed her personality and was more happy than unhappy with it. She had an inflexible desire for the "old Jay" or the stereotypical, dominant male fantasy character she believed she needed. Jay, on the other hand, was maturing and adjusting to his illness and his own personality type. He was more in need of an equal partner with whom he could share his love, his responsibilities, and his disease without guilt.

A person with multiple sclerosis often feels ashamed that he is "sick" because our society puts such a high value on the "well" role. He may be dependent on others in some aspects of his life, while at the same time resent them for the care they provide. The anger directed at a caregiver in such situations is partially a projection of the anger the person feels toward himself for his illness. We think so much of self-reliance that feeling comfortable relying on others, or being relied upon, is extremely problematic.

"I hate having to be cared for," declares Marty. "Every time I wake up to a day in my wheelchair, I just fill with rage. I was an athlete in college. I played tennis or squash almost every day. I was active. I was fit. I was proud of what I could do. And then to be knocked down by this damn thing and thrown into a wheelchair is almost more than I can bear sometimes.

"But that's not the worst part of it. The worst is having to have Mary, my wife, help me in and out of the chair. Or push me uphill when we're out someplace. I want to do more for myself. I'm so angry at what's become of me, I feel so helpless that I don't even feel like doing what I can do. I guess Mary gets the brunt of my anger. I feel she either is not there when I need her or else is hovering around too much asking me what I need. I guess I'm so angry I feel there's nothing she can do right."

"Marty," Mary says right back, "is one royal pain. I get so angry at him and his games. We all have problems. He thinks he's the only one that's ever had to stop doing what he loves. Of course, I feel terrible for him. He's always done whatever he could by himself. And now he has to have other people help with some of his most private needs. He rages at me that I'm more a burden than a help, but I guess I was born with the patience of a saint, and I do love the man, so I put up with a lot of his nonsense.

"But I tell you, he'd better get his act together. Even a saint would get worn down by his crankiness. I've wanted him to see a counselor with me, but he refuses because that would be admitting he has a problem that he needs help with, which, of course, is exactly the point. I tell him strong men can ask for help, weak men need to feel they're always strong, but he just won't do it. Unfortunately, if he doesn't he may lose more than his health."

It is vital for two people in a relationship to work out the complex dynamics that are present when one is ill or less able. Sooner or later every marriage or other long-term commitment enters phases, often alternating, of care and dependency. The words "through sickness and in health," spoken in most marriage ceremonies, both implicitly and explicitly tell a couple that there will be times when mutual aid and comfort will be needed. So it can be of enormous help to understand more fully and consciously the accompanying issues of guilt and anger. This is one area where thoughtful professional counseling can be of particularly good use.

"David was not too keen on my mother's coming to live with us after my father died," Thalassa remembers. "Our children were old enough that we were able to be more independent, and we were looking forward to traveling. Both of his parents were still alive and he didn't understand the need I felt to ensure that my mother felt secure and wanted. I have a brother and a sister, but they are not as well off as we and I felt an obligation, as well as a desire, to take care of her."

David picks up the discussion. "Thalassa had always managed the relationships with both sets of parents and I just assumed she would be able to handle this just as successfully, without allowing too much overlap onto our family's lives. Looking back, I can see how selfish I was. I feel bad that I gave her such a hard time, even if I had not become ill with M.S."

"My mother had not been with us for more than a year," Thalassa continues, "when David's symptoms appeared. He was affected pretty badly rather quickly, and all of a sudden I had two people I thought I had to take care of. I became very anxious and depressed with what seemed like an overwhelming turn of events. My mother was still getting over the death of my father and the move into our house. The days of taking care of two babies now looked invitingly easy. I started going to a counselor to help me deal with the situation and my feelings of panic that I would be overrun by events."

"It became clear that Thalassa's mother's being there was more a blessing than the burden I feared," David relates. "When Thalassa would go to her therapy appointments, her mother and I would be left alone with each other and we could no longer avoid talking about some of the issues we had let get between us. Our concern for Thalassa was greater than our individual concerns. Her mother's spirits rallied and she began to be much more helpful around the house and with the children, which freed Thalassa to have more time for herself and for us. All of us learned something about love, that's for sure."

"My therapist was wonderful," Thalassa remembers. "He was very appreciative of what I felt were my obligations toward others. I was afraid I would find a counselor who stressed my personal needs and growth before my concern for my family. That would have split me cruelly. He supported my sense of self as being inseparable from my relationships with the important people in my life.

"But he also helped me to recognize that there had to be some reciprocity from others, that it was okay to expect my mother and David, despite her grief and his illness, to help. I could not do it all alone, but we could manage it together. My memories of family meetings with my mother and David and our sharing of sorrow and compassion are unforgettably warm and at the very center of my being."

Coping with a spouse's or companion's multiple sclerosis can mean major changes in friendship, career, and leisure activities for the healthy one. "When Cynthia got M.S.," reports Darrell, "her illness progressed so rapidly that I knew right away that there would be differences in the way she lived her life and what we did together, but I had little idea how much my personal activities would be affected.

"I had to do more around the house—cleaning, grocery shopping, cooking, laundry—and I started out quite enthusiastically. I was going to be Superdad: work, take care of home, chauffeur the kids. Fortunately, I think, I don't have rigid sex role ideas, so I wasn't bothered by doing 'women's work' kind of stuff. But after six months or so it lost its glamour, and I began to see that this wasn't an experiment in role-changing, it was my life!

"I began to get snappy whenever anyone asked what I was cooking for that night's meal. I was wondering to myself whether Cynthia couldn't manage to do at least a little more around the house. The adventure of looking through cookbooks for great meals in sixty minutes became the chore of finding something that everyone would eat without complaining.

"What really started to depress me, however, was that the time I spent around the house meant less time for golf and tennis, which were my releases from the pressures of work. I was taking more of my work home with me and I must have become a pretty cranky, old man to live with. Up to now, my way of dealing with tough situations was to joke about them, but I was around my buddies much less than before.

"All this time Cynthia was telling me to get some help for cleaning or let my mother do the shopping, which she had offered to do," Darrell continues. "But I insisted that I could do it all and, more than that, I should do it all. One night, after a hectic dinner when I was angry with everyone, the kids and Cynthia confronted me, asked me what I was trying to prove, and announced that they would prefer to eat crackers and sleep in dirty sheets than have me running around like a madman making life miserable for all. After that I came to my senses. We've organized things, set some priorities, and although I'm obviously doing more than before, we're all much more relaxed."

What was Darrell trying to prove and what were the changes that Cynthia and he made that allowed him to cope more successfully with the life-style changes required by her illness? First, Darrell heroically attempted to keep the home running as it had prior to Cynthia's illness. He pretended that Cynthia's illness was merely an inconvenience, not an obstacle, to their continuing with their former domestic patterns.

In addition, Darrell's taking on of extra burdens that he could have handed to others was in some ways a compensation for the guilt he felt at remaining able-bodied while his wife was ill. Darrell's exhausting efforts represented, as well, a wish to undo the feelings of betrayal he had for failing to protect Cynthia from suffering and hardship. It is important to understand that there are seldom single motivations for thoughts, feelings, and actions, particularly in circumstances as complex and difficult as these.

"Talking with a therapist," Darrell says, "helped me to see that although my feelings of guilt for Cynthia's illness were normal, I was in no way responsible for her illness, nor could my frantic efforts around the house heal her. It was very painful for me to acknowledge that our life-style would be different and that there was little I could do to maintain it at its pre-illness status. In fact, my actions prevented us from making the necessary adjustments.

"Our therapist also pointed out the difference between life-style and 'life values.' Although our style of living would change, our values need not alter. In fact, Cynthia's M.S. forced me to reconsider what was most important to me: my career, or my children and my marriage. I had to think about that seriously. I knew that if I was not clear about that choice, as soon as things got rough I would bail out. And I have made my choice—for Cynthia and our children, marriage and family. I gave up style for value—a good trade, it seems to me."

Both Darrell and Cynthia also made a decision to relax their standards of housekeeping. They expected their children to pitch in more, although they did not shift the burden of maintaining the home to them. The couple also accepted more readily their parents' offers of help even though it meant that how their parents did things did not always match their preferences. Gradually, Darrell and Cynthia became less rigid in the expectations they held for themselves and more tolerant toward their parents.

Darrell had worked very hard as a young adult and husband and father to create firm boundaries between himself and his parents. This separation was necessary so he could develop as his own person. Now that he felt more secure about himself and his ability to meet adversity, he could more easily reach out to his parents and in-laws and make good use of their offers of help.

Darrell became more conscious and accepting of the network of shared dependencies and care of which all relationships—marriages and families—are made. That he could not do it all by himself, nor that anyone expected it of him or thought it possible of him, was a welcome and humbling realization. From that knowledge, Darrell gained the strength to ask for help when he needed it and to be more compassionate toward those who, like himself, he now realized, needed support. As a result of Cynthia's illness and the changes Darrell made, he no longer asked "for whom the bell tolls."

An additional complication of M.S. for a couple is the different and often more difficult process of decision making. A natural uneasiness about possible future problems is compounded by the unpredictable mobility of the M.S. person. Joanne was diagnosed with M.S. at the same time she and Rolfe (her husband of four years) had been going through a fertility program to conceive their first child. This program included a support group, frequent doctor appointments, and regular monthly checkups that were continued at home.

Their commitment to the program and desire for natural childbirth was total until the potential effects of her diagnosis were realized. Because they have a comfortable, respectful relationship with each other, they were able to explore their potential as parents. They addressed, step by step, all the possible complications that could arise in Joanne's condition during pregnancy and early child-rearing years. They were very clear about the full partnership childcare requires.

"My husband is my partner. He is also my best friend," Joanne told her support group while revealing her final decision. "He has agreed that, if necessary, as soon as the baby is born, he or she can be handed over to him for as much care as necessary. We've agreed to share it all—job changes, house moves, housework— everything."

Rolfe sums up his philosophy of married life this way: "Joanne and I are in this together. The baby will be both of ours, but that does not represent a complete change. After all, her M.S. is both of ours, too. We live it together."

Making an important decision during a time of crisis can generate a great deal of stress and often result in choices that are much regretted later. Sometimes, however, the anxiety a couple feels at the time of a diagnosis or exacerbation is such that they attempt to relieve it by taking some kind of action that they hope will take care of the problem. Often, a couple will fight with each other over whether to do this or that as a way of avoiding confronting the strong emotions each has about the illness.

Jane, for example, was diagnosed with M.S. just as she and her husband were about to begin a home remodeling project. She had few symptoms, was minimally disabled, and the course of her disease had stabilized. When she learned of her illness, she became very confused and fearful. "The only person I knew who may have had M.S. was someone from my childhood neighborhood who was in a wheelchair," Jane says. "I told Michael we just had to call off the project or else change everything. I wanted a bathroom big enough for a wheelchair and to bring all our washing appliances up from the basement. The next day I wanted to sell our colonial-style house and buy a ranch or split level.

"Michael and I had battles over whether or not to remodel, whether to stay where we were, or whether to purchase another place. We spent an enormous amount of energy fighting. We never stopped to ask what M.S. was, what kind of future I could expect, or what it would mean for our life together. I see now that our wanting to make big decisions *now* was our way of denying together my, our, illness."

Decisions about residence, employment, children, travel, vacations, and marriage may have to be made, but they don't usually have to be resolved immediately. Many issues can be addressed without haste, with attention to what a couple wants, rather than running from what they want to avoid. Many couples find, however, that it is easier to argue about these relatively concrete problems than to come to terms with the unpredictability of multiple sclerosis.

It is quite common for one spouse or partner to grapple with and face the meaning of the diagnosis of M.S. more quickly than the other. Typically, it is the partner without the disease who moves along the path of adjustment, and the ill person who plays catch-up. That two people are not in step with each other in the complex process is quite expected. That the more "advanced" partner may become impatient is understandable as well.

"Being out of synch" can provide added stress to the marital and family system. The spouse who listens empathetically to her ill partner may find no similar understanding. She knows where he's coming from, but he seems ignorant of her own inner travail. In whom can she confide? She feels guilty sharing the secrets of symptoms that he is embarrassed to admit.

"I used to cry myself to sleep on the nights when I wasn't too tired or numb to feel anything," offers Alice. "It seemed as if all I heard from anyone was 'How's Richie?' 'Is Richie feeling okay?' 'How is Richie handling his M.S.?' No one asked me how was I handling Richie's handling of his M.S. Because the truth was, although I never told anyone, that neither one of us was handling anything very well.

"Although he gave the appearance of not complaining and shrugging off any worries about it, the fact is that Richie either denied what was wrong with him or between us, or he'd become depressed when he was alone with me. I felt trapped. If I told anyone what was really going on, I would be accused of telling secrets. If I confronted Richie, he would tell me I was worrying too much, it was his illness and he would manage. And of course, he wasn't managing.

"I knew that there was no quick way to come to terms with M.S. either for Richie or me or our marriage, but he didn't seem to want to make the effort it would take. I suggested therapy or talking with friends, anything. I told him he was slowly pushing himself off a cliff, and that he wouldn't be able to get back up. But he would have none of it. I was paying for his inability to confront his own fears.

"I was becoming very depressed. I felt that maybe I wasn't giving Richie what he needed, that I didn't understand his needs enough, that maybe I was pushing him too hard to come to terms with being sick. At work, people noticed that I was preoccupied, but no one approached me to ask why—and I'm sure that if they had I would have shrugged them off because I would have felt that I was betraying Richie's privacy.

"Finally, Richie's neurologist's office called one day to verify an appointment and I asked if the doctor could speak to me. When he came on the phone I poured everything out to him. The next time I drove Richie over for the appointment, the doctor asked me to come into the office, too. He suggested we see a social worker to talk about any adjustment problems. I made an appointment that Richie refused to keep, but I went.

"I was so happy to finally have someone to share my feelings with. We urged Richie to come in and talk, but he still refused. My worker encouraged me to talk to people. She said I was not betraying Richie by talking about my feelings, fears, and needs. I talked to his mother and sister. I talked to friends. They were glad to support me. They encouraged Richie to talk, but he pushed everyone away.

"Eventually, after two years, I separated from Richie. I left the door open to come back if he could get his act together. His relatives and our friends supported me. Richie just could not face his life. It's sad, very sad. But I could no longer let my life drift away as he had done with his. I hope one day he'll wake up to what he's lost and what he still has to live for."

Seeking professional counseling at a time like this may be very beneficial. Many people imagine that they should be able to handle "normal" crises, like illness, by themselves. The fact that they are adjusting satisfactorily and supporting their stricken partner often leads them to forget their own need for appreciation, encouragement, and a sympathetic ear.

A relationship that includes chronic illness is a trying yet potentially rewarding one. The firmer the ties and the more flexible the partners before a crisis occurs, the more resilient and helpful the alliance, both individually and in concert, after the diagnosis. The opportunity to love another in health and in sickness is a great gift. To assume that life offers us only what we want when we want it is a grotesque and, ultimately, self-defeating fantasy. Responding to what life presents with the fullness of humanity we can muster is the alchemical secret. The capacity to make and maintain enduring commitments with other people, weathering circumstances that fate and accident toss up, is true maturity. Multiple sclerosis provides an occasion for couples to take steps together beyond either romance or despair toward wisdom and serenity.

✦ 3 ✦

What Is Happening to Us?

CHANGE AND TRANSITION is a normal part of every family's life cycle. The addition and departure of family members is a process all families undergo. Babies are born, children begin school, mothers enter or return to the workplace, young people encounter puberty and soon depart for college. Grandparents age, husband and wife confront mid-life choices, death visits older loved ones. These are some of the typical events that most families experience, adapt to, and learn from.

Although these transition points, as family therapists know, can be more or less difficult for different families, they are common enough. Thus, people who work with families describe these stages as normative. On the other hand, less-anticipated crises impact upon many families. Chronic illness, accidents, sudden unemployment, drug and alcohol abuse, separation and divorce, natural disaster, unexpected death are some of the stressors that may yield hardship or, indeed, catastrophe for a family.

How a particular family responds to normative or catastrophic events is influenced by several factors, including the family's existing financial and psychological resources, ongoing demands with which the family members must currently cope, and the definition the family places upon the event. Families that are willing to confront problems directly and communicate how best to meet them are likely to sustain and serve their members better over the long term.

Ben and Carol were understandably shocked and dismayed when Ben's three years of symptoms were finally diagnosed as a result of multiple sclerosis. Although Ben was at the time minimally disabled, no physician wanted to assure the couple that his health would remain unimpaired. He was unable to ride a bike or walk unassisted for more than a block, and there was no way of knowing whether more severe exacerbations were likely.

"Ben and I decided we would meet this thing head-on, and the best way to do that for us was to talk and talk some more," says Carol. "We had a good marriage. I was able to talk with Ben about my fears and concerns, and although, like many men, Ben was not as forthcoming about his own anxieties, he listened to me. I guess I was able to articulate for him what I thought he might be going through. If he disagreed with my hunches about his experience, he would correct me. I know it may not be the ideal way of 'sharing,' but it was one that worked for us. I read somewhere that men have feelings and the words for feelings, but they have problems connecting words with feelings. That might be true, but Ben and I didn't let that get in our way.

"After we talked about the feelings we had about Ben's illness and ourselves, we made different boxes for Ben and me individually, our marriage, our children, our relatives and friends, our work, our leisure, our finances. Then we made a list in each box of the ways we thought M.S. could affect our lives. The next step was to begin to think about what we could do to deal with those difficulties.

"We did this over several weeks," Carol goes on. "At the same time we talked about our children and our parents and what to tell each. We didn't just pick up the phone and tell everybody the diagnosis. We didn't know enough about M.S. to be able to answer all the questions they might ask or to respond to all the fears they might have.

"So the next thing we did was make a list of all the questions we had or other people might have about M.S. Then we wrote down the answers we knew and made it a point to speak with Ben's neurologist or call the M.S. Society to get the information we needed. They were enormously helpful. Only then did we feel comfortable letting people know Ben's diagnosis. I know that most people may not have the desire or the discipline to use our approach, but it worked for us better than we imagined.

"Both our parents were initially upset that we had not told them as soon as we knew the diagnosis, but once we explained why we had delayed and were able to answer all their questions, they were relieved. Ben's parents, in particular, are quite emotional, but because we could address their anxieties directly with facts and doctor's words, they could approach the situation more calmly. We didn't hold anything back. We answered as best we could. If we didn't know something, we said we'd find out and we did.

"With our children, seven and ten years old, we decided they did not need to know more than they were capable of asking. They could see that Ben was not able to do as much with them as before in terms of ball playing and bike riding. We let them know that Ben had something called multiple sclerosis by talking a little about it with each other while we were all at the dinner table. That was enough for them to ask what M.S. was. We answered them simply and we let them know they could ask anything they wanted to know. I'm sure they got the message that M.S. was something they could talk about, and occasionally they'd ask a question or say something. They saw literature from the M.S. Society around the house and newsletters and such.

"Again," Carol concludes, "I'm not sure if we did the right thing or the best thing, but we feel it worked for us. We felt open and honest with everybody, not necessarily bringing up issues, but always ready and available to address them. And if the proof is in the pudding, I'd say we did all right. Our kids feel as safe and confident about their family and the future as they ever did and, at the same time, they know perfectly well their dad has an illness that prevents him from doing some of the things other kids' fathers can do. But he can still talk with them, read to them, play games with them, and, most importantly, love them. Ben's physical disability doesn't impair his fathering ability."

There is no question that a diagnosis of multiple sclerosis is a traumatic occurrence for any family—parents, children, and extended relations included. How information is shared throughout the family system may set a pattern of functional or dysfunctional coping for a long time to come. The trust and confidence in each other that an individual or family needs during periods of stress can be seriously compromised during this early stage.

Unfortunately, a family's best intentions are sometimes poorly thought out and go awry. Elaine Gold was diagnosed with M.S. at age thirty-two, after she had lost control of her right leg and fell. She was then the mother of a two-year-old child. Her family, with the backing of their family doctor, decided not to reveal the diagnosis to Elaine.

This decision may not have reflected what Elaine would have wanted, but may have solved a problem for her family: how to relate to Elaine. It is, therefore, important to focus on the interaction of these family members to understand how their duplicity appeared to be a logical progression of past events, and not due to M.S. alone. This family's psychological resources were reduced prior to a diagnosis of a chronic disease. M.S. merely continued the dysfunctional pattern.

The Gold family consists of a mother and father and two sisters, two years apart. Elaine, the older sister, was considered a "problem" for as long as her parents could remember. Her sister, Gladys, had a strong bond with their mother. Relatives would always comment on how these two "were naturals with each other." They looked alike and seemed to like the same things. In contrast, Elaine had her own curiosity about the world. She would not accept anyone's prior experience; she had to discover things on her own. Her ideas, tastes, and goals were often different from her mother's. As a result, her mother would reinforce Gladys's ideas and sharply contradict Elaine's. Elaine had to fight for her right to express herself. As a result, as Gladys became the "good daughter" who was easy to please, Elaine became the one labeled "difficult" and "headstrong." At first, Mrs. Gold assumed that when Elaine disagreed with her she was being aggressive and negative. She did not appreciate the fact that Elaine was merely trying to assert herself.

As a very young child, Elaine's basic goal was to define her place in the family, and to be recognized as an individual. When she tried to choose her own clothes and to dress herself in the morning, Mrs. Gold would chide her deliberate, reflective approach. "I'm in a hurry," her mother would insist, "let me do this for you." When Elaine would attempt to assist her mother around the house, her mother would respond, "Whenever you do something I always have to do it over again. It's easier to do things myself than to leave them to you." Elaine soon learned to feel most important while she and her mother were in a power struggle. And her mother never learned how to positively reinforce her older daughter by giving her time to fulfill her responsibilities in order to enlist her cooperation for the future. Gladys, watching Elaine's difficulties in pleasing their mother, tried to mimic her mother's approach to things. She emulated her mother's gestures, cleaning habits, scheduling of tasks. "It was easier to do things like Mom," she explained to Elaine several years later. "I certainly didn't want to get into trouble the way you did." Even as an adult, reflecting upon these difficult years, Elaine could not smile on hearing her younger sister's reasoning. "You're right, as usual," she assured Gladys in a rueful manner. "I can't remember a time that Mom and I were not arguing about something."

As Elaine matured into adolescence, her choice of activities contrasted even more strongly with her mother's. She was positively reinforced by her close friends, and so began to be more influenced by their dress, actions, and conversation. She became more outspoken against her mother, who found less time for Elaine as she found more time for Gladys. Gladys began to take tennis lessons with Mrs. Gold, and soon the two became partners in mother-daughter tournaments. The community marveled at how alike they were on the court. Elaine never did watch a match. Her mother used to insist to her friends, "This is yet another example of her rejection. It is not as if Elaine has been too busy to watch our matches, she just chooses to hang out with her friends."

It soon became easier for the family to ignore Elaine. Her father describes those difficult years: "I felt helpless. It was simpler for me to stay out of the arguments. If I sided with Elaine, then my wife would become angry; if I sided with her mother against her, then Elaine would become more oppositional and just leave the house. It was as if Elaine expected me to be quiet and leave them alone to fight it out." When asked about how he felt about Gladys, Mr. Gold would smile. "She was such an easy, likable kid. We three got along so well when Elaine wasn't around. Gladys never disagreed. You know," he would marvel, "even as a married woman living in a neighboring state, she still phones us every day. And Elaine? We're lucky to hear from her once every other week."

Elaine attended college quite far from home and succeeded in cutting herself off from her family for most of the school year. "When I came home for vacations," she readily explains, "we would be careful not to discuss anything controversial. I had my life and they had theirs. Though Gladys would talk to my mother about her courses, clothes, and consult her about her social plans, I would make my own decisions, and soon they stopped questioning me. They continued to avoid dealing with me about anything serious."

Multiple sclerosis symptoms threatened to destroy the careful web of noncommunication to which this family had adjusted. The Gold family arbitrarily decided not to deal with the illness. They never learned how to be supportive of Elaine. And so, they explained to their family doctor, "for her own good, they would protect her from this for as long as they could."

"My fatigue, balance problems, and difficulties with the summer heat and humidity," Elaine remembers, "were all treated as 'nerve problems' that rest would heal. I guess my family thought I'd rather think I was crazy than ill," she adds with some anger.

For ten years, Elaine continued to be puzzled by her abrupt change from good health to weakness. It wasn't until she was visiting her sister and needed the services of a doctor for a sudden loss of strength and coordination that she learned the truth. She asked the doctor what had happened and he responded without awareness of the family's masquerade, "Well, this has to be expected when you have M.S."

Elaine memorized the two letters that had no meaning for her at that time and asked her sister what M.S. might stand for. Reluctantly, Gladys told her the story.

Furious that she had been lied to, Elaine left for home immediately and demanded a family meeting with her parents, sister, brother-in-law, and, even, estranged husband in attendance. All admitted to knowing the diagnosis. "It was for your own good" was the unanimous explanation for their deception.

It took Elaine many months with a counselor and a number of soul-searching talks with close friends to finally realize that her family's denial was due to their inability to deal with her illness, as well as illness in general.

"I was angry and bitter for a long time," states Elaine. "I wondered whether they might have been right to protect me. But eventually I saw that they did not have faith in my strength. I could have coped with the news a good deal better than they did by denying me the respect for my adulthood and the truth." Elaine's family's collusion led her to doubt herself and, unfortunately, lose the opportunities for support they might otherwise have provided.

The reaction of a family such as Elaine's is not simply a denial of the fact of illness. It represents, as well, an attempt to avoid the disorganization and changes in the family that admission of a crisis would bring. By not allowing Elaine to face the reality of her M.S. and her own individual response, the family cuts down on the number and complexity of adjustments it must make. Over the short term, this family's response to crisis and stress was an attempt to keep the existing family system intact—dysfunctional though it was.

Just as some families, like Elaine's, tend to "hush up" unpleasant news, other families cope with difficult events by spreading their anxiety around. The concern that family members show each other in such a system may cloak a family's obsession with potential negative consequences.

"I speak to my mother each week," Joan explains, "but our conversations are always the same. Since she learned of my M.S. diagnosis two years ago, she attempts more and more to smother me. She always asks the same questions and she asks them as if I'm hiding the truth from her. She thinks she has to confront me like a detective to find out what's really going on. 'Are you getting enough rest? Do your husband and the children help out?' Of course, the more she asks me like that, the less I want to tell her."

Just as Elaine's family continued to undermine her by refusing to share the truth of her condition with her,

Joan's mother treats her like a child by acting as if Joan is not able to take care of herself and recognize her own needs. Two different styles of reacting to stress in the family—one underinvolved, the other overinvolved—yet neither respects the autonomy of the person who is ill. The result in both cases is further restriction of communication and, as a result, an inability to call on others for support.

Joan and her mother were stuck in the same roles they had when Joan was a young, inexperienced child. During those years, her mother's responsibility was to care for her. She accomplished this in a didactic manner. It was difficult for Joan's mother to alter her approach, to consider her daughter as an adult, though in time this, too, was accomplished. Joan recalls when she had to refuse her mother a key to her home, shortly after she and Dan were married. "She was furious, and insulted," Joan relates, "to think that she could not enter our home whenever she wished, whether we were home or not." Mrs. Smith had difficulty understanding the boundaries that Joan wanted to establish between her mother and herself, between generations.

Another difficult situation arose when Joan began to space her phone calls to her mother. "Instead of phoning her each day," Joan explains, "I would be in touch with her only on a weekly basis." Mrs. Smith was insulted that her older daughter appeared to need her less, but to this, too, she had had to adjust. In contrast, Joan's siblings lived in the same town as their mother and continued to consult her on a daily basis for all of their needs. Instead of noting their dependent, immature approach, Mrs. Smith remained flattered at her other children's needs. She continued to overinvolve herself in their affairs, refusing to recognize how inappropriate her infantilization of Joan's sisters was for their age and maturity expectations.

"I remained hesitant to share my M.S. diagnosis with my mother," Joan recalls. "I was convinced she would overreact, which she did. It seemed as if she always focused on how situations would affect her, never realizing how the diagnosis could change my self-image, if I allowed this to happen." By refusing her mother's desire to infantilize her, Joan remained independent and mature.

Mrs. Smith, in contrast, quickly announced to the family, "Joan has proven to be less strong than she thought she was. She is really sick now, and certainly will need my help. She will soon appreciate what a devoted mother she has; I'll be glad to assist her whenever necessary."

As a result, Joan often tries to minimize her symptoms to her mother. Even when she would appreciate help with chores, she refuses to admit this to Mrs. Smith. "I could not stand her handwringing and worrying aloud," Joan admits. The mother and daughter are then caught in a negative loop, or tug-of-war, situation. Mrs. Smith is overanxious to be of assistance to her "poor, sick daughter," partially to satisfy herself about her usefulness. Joan remains anxious to avoid regressing to a dependency on her mother that she has struggled hard to avoid. "I enjoy my adult status," she explains, "and refuse to give it up.

"I find that now I'm really reluctant to let my mother know how I'm feeling or if I'm worried," confides Joan. "I think when I was younger that was my way of dealing with what I felt was my mother's intrusiveness. She's still like that, so now both my husband and I are starting to keep information to ourselves so it won't 'leak' to my mother. If that happens it gets spread around to the family and her friends. I'm sure my mother needs to feel she knows everything in order to maintain some control over her emotions and situations, but she doesn't realize how that concern is getting her the opposite of what she wants. We're shutting her out."

"We've talked about what we could do to help calm Joan's mother's anxiety," says Dan, Joan's husband. "We tried giving her booklets from the M.S. Society, but she doesn't read them. We sat down with her and told her all about M.S. and said we'd answer any questions, but she couldn't stay focused. I guess we just need to be careful about how much we tell her—too much and she gets very overanxious, too little and she keeps pushing for more. It's taken us a while, but I think we've finally found a somewhat happy medium. It's certainly a strain we don't need."

Families that have established clear communications about individual and group accomplishments and needs are better able to cope when a crisis or new strain appears. When Rose heard her diagnosis, she patiently explained to her doctor, "You don't understand. I'm too busy to be sick. I'm already playing checkers with time in order to get everything done at home and at work."

Because Rose had so much confidence in her family's ability to function under adversity, she declined to give up or modify any of her roles. She was determined not to ask for help. "When I learned I had M.S., all I could think about was who was going to drive Joey to Little League? If I were too tired to cook, how would my family eat? I probably overemphasized how much I was responsible for, but I didn't like thinking about all the compromises the family might have to make. I felt so guilty.

"I never did think of asking for help until the children and my husband scolded me for not letting them in on my silent thoughts. They said I talked a lot less with them, and it was true. I wanted quiet around me so I wouldn't be interrupted in my thinking about my situation and how I could manage it all. I admitted to them that if I talked about problems or asked for help, I'd feel I was complaining.

"Frank [Rose's husband] got quite angry. He said he was very hurt that he wasn't involved in my worries as well as my plans for the children. He thought it was important for him and me and for the children to all pitch in and help. He was a husband and father, too, he said, not just Mr. Paycheck. 'It isn't just you that has multiple sclerosis,' he said. 'It's something we all live with and we'll all take care of together.' "

Rose's family knew something was wrong when their typically sharing mother had become closemouthed. They responded with real concern and offers to help so she could do as much as she was able and, at the same time, know there were others she could rely on. Rose's M.S. served as a catalyst for the family to reexamine its priorities and scheduling and to develop a support structure of family and friends that could help everyone, including Rose, have their needs met.

When family members listen to each other, self-blame, guilt, denial, and anger are minimized and replaced by positive mutual support. Francine's family, for example, continued to respond to her with respect after her diagnosis. Her positive attitude permeated the family's interactions. "Life," she explains, "is like a checkbook. Yesterday is a canceled check; tomorrow is a promissory note; but today is cash in hand. How can anyone waste that fistful of dollars?

"When I found out I had M.S., I'm sure we went through a lot of confusion, self-pity, and refusing to believe it could happen to us. But we kept talking.

I think that's what made it work out okay for our family. Right away we knew that this illness was *our* illness and *our* challenge. We recognized that we needed each other and as a unit we would go through this together.

"I believe," Francine states with conviction, "that I'm a person first, and an M.S. patient second, particularly during an attack." For her Mother's Day celebration, Francine received a cane as a gift. "It was so funny and outrageous. The children had all of their friends sign it with original sayings and unusual designs. They said that as I walked, I would take all their thoughts with me. I was so touched by their caring.

"Sometimes I feel overprotected," Francine confides to her close friends, "and then we have a family meeting and figure out where to go from there." Because this family is so overtly committed to each other, the lines of communication are always open. "It's not easy. M.S. is such a trying disease with its ups and downs, attacks and remissions, that we are always readjusting. But we have to be patient—and positive. And we'll make it all work out together. I'll always accept their help when I need it. They all know that and remain supportive. In some ways, my M.S. has been a constant reminder of what our family is and what it's for."

It's clear that one major influence upon a family's adjustment is how the fact of the diagnosis and a chronic illness is defined. How serious is it? Is it likely to be viewed as catastrophic in impact—a tragic omen of the family's demise? Or is it seen as a challenge to be faced with courage and unity?

Families that accept a narrow and, ultimately, unrealistic interpretation of life that has no place for sorrow, pain, loss, and the unexpected will have a very tortuous time attempting to adjust to unwanted demands.

On the other hand, families that are conscious of both the fragility and the tenacity of life, that sense the tragic undertow that may flow beneath our current enjoyment, that realize the joy and sense of joined purpose that can arise from sharing another's happiness and distress will fare much better in times of trouble and need.

The Stanleys are such a family. Colin is a business executive and Ginny is a social worker. Both shared a commitment to what they called "good works"— devoting a significant portion of their spare time to helping out with community programs and social action projects for those financially less fortunate than they.

"From when our children were young," says Colin, "we felt it important that they develop a feeling for reaching out and offering a hand to others. In many ways, our family's good fortune has been a matter of birth and luck. We feel we have an obligation to others. When Ginny was diagnosed with multiple sclerosis it didn't lessen our interest in helping. In fact, it reinforced our belief in the mystery of life's outcomes. Why are some people afflicted with illness and others blessed with good health? Why are some rich and others poor?"

Ginny continues, "When I became ill, we were determined to use the damn disease as a way of standing up to life's pain. We were helpless to control the M.S., but we could control how we responded to it. By not changing how we related to our own family, with intimacy and sharing, and to others, with support and empathy, we could transform some of the private pain of our lives and be of some use to others.

"My illness was a turning point for our children. Their best instincts were often overwhelmed by the social indifference around them. It was easy for toys and stereos and fashion to become more important than hunger and homelessness and peace. But when they saw me in a wheelchair and saw that my friends and family offered and shared so much, they realized how close each of us was to needing help at some time.

"I guess they woke up. They became much more pleasant and, in a fundamental way, more serious people. They gained a new and more realistic perspective of life that I hope they hold onto as they grow older. It will certainly make their lives easier and happier in the long run. I get so mad at people who think life is supposed to be some perpetual, sunny day."

Although it is often true that a family that is uncomfortable communicating about emotionally charged issues has problems dealing with the diagnosis of a chronic illness, the individual with the disease can reinforce and amplify those difficulties. James prided himself on his masculine self-image. No one had ever seen him shed a tear. He was a self-made man; he attained success without the benefit of anyone's sponsorship or any higher education. He was married only a few months when he was diagnosed as having M.S. His wife wanted to be supportive and share this experience with him. He immediately shut her out. His children from another marriage sought private time with him. He was angry and defensive about accepting their "sympathy."

"I don't want anyone to feel sorry for me," James insisted. "I can make it alone. No one will ever hear me asking for help." James's fatigue and constant limping embarrassed him. "I will never get handicap plates on my car," he admonished anyone who suggested it. "I'm not any different from the rest of the world."

Nevertheless, despite and, in many ways, due to his maladaptive coping strategies and his multiple sclerosis, James's world changed considerably. His emotional swings from the illness were compounded considerably by his anger, fear, and general hostility. His home environment became more uncomfortable each year and a solid and harmonious adjustment could not be accomplished. Despite his stated attempts of not over-burdening his family with his illness, James's own denial and discomfort with M.S. were responsible for a dysfunctional resolution of this, in truth, family problem.

James refused to alter his self-image as an athletic, healthy male whose body-building goals represented his chief objective for building self-esteem. He spent considerable energy spinning fantasies that were, at this time in his life, impossible to achieve. If James had spent more time using the power of creative imagination to focus on what was possible for him, he would have been less depressed and more able to integrate the fact of his illness into his self-concept.

To do this does not mean he had to give up hope or settle for rather weak expectations. This task does require, however, the art and courage of recognizing limits and stretching to their boundaries. By tempering his wishes with realism, James could have helped family members to cease "spinning their wheels" emotionally while they waited for him to catch up to their adjustment.

Instead, James continued to be depressed and continued to disturb his family with his anger, bitterness, and rage. He obsessed over wishes for himself that remained impossible to realize rather than picture himself accomplishing more likely goals. For example, he never considered learning any new skills. His legs were stiff, but his arms were unencumbered by the disease. He could still work out to strengthen his upper body, but "it wasn't worth it."

His children drifted further and further away, repelled

by his negative comments and despairing attitude about life. They could not tolerate his constant criticism of their activities, friends, and dress. His wife no longer looked forward to coming home after work. He no longer allowed his family, nor were they interested in trying, to distract him from his depression.

This couple never divorced, but only because of James's wife's strong commitment to the concept of marriage and family. She did, however, seek out a male colleague at work in whom to confide about the unsatisfactory relationship she was having with James because of his moods.

Unfortunately, James became very angry and even more bitter when he learned of his wife's new confidant. He constantly blamed M.S. for his marital problems. In this case, however, James's personality, poor adjustment, and lack of flexibility were more to blame for his family's problems than was his multiple sclerosis. He probably would have reacted in much the same manner to any normative or unexpected crisis. He may well have attempted to counter his normal aging by living among past glories and wishing for impossible youth. James could have benefited from assistance in how to control his own negativism. Although his illness was an act of fate, to seek help was not beyond his choosing.

Blaming a disease, like blaming someone else for your own misfortune, simply leads to more negative consequences. The anger and bitterness James felt about his M.S. was extended toward his wife and children. Whenever anyone challenged him about the hopelessness he felt or suggested that his emotional crisis was not a product of his illness, he would announce, "I know my disease best." The children took him at his word and developed equally poor attitudes.

James's teenage son refused to entertain any idea of

driving a car that had handicap plates. Eighteen-year-old Mark insisted that "kids think the person behind the wheel must be different, queer with those plates on. I don't want everyone to look at me, expecting me to look like him." Instead of trying to understand where Mark's comments came from, James talked resentfully about his "mean kid who's too selfish to understand me." He failed to notice that Mark's words were simply reflections of his own.

Most children respond quite well to the painful reality of a parent with multiple sclerosis. Like adults, however, they do have their own anxieties, fears, and concerns that thoughtful parents would do well to address. While the wish to spare children the struggle of coming to terms with a parent's diagnosis may be understandable, it usually only delays the process of adjustment.

We do not mean to suggest that a child should be told everything about a parent's illness and be expected to be capable of dealing with it all. Rather, there are issues that children and adults can disclose and discuss to create a context for open and honest communication among family members. A child's sense of trust and "approachability" with a parent around any concern is the foundation for making M.S. a positive family challenge instead of an overwhelming catastrophe.

Children often notice the symptoms of multiple sclerosis before their parents have been diagnosed. Fatigue, weakness of arms and legs, stumbling, vision problems, incontinence may all be observed and commented upon by children, who then may be given explanations for these difficulties.

Once the true diagnosis is known, they can be given more accurate information. Most children (including teens) want to know what is happening to their mother or father and how it will affect them. But, like adults, they may fear knowing because what they learn may be awful.

They also may feel quite sad and helpless about the illness and fantasize that if they are "good" or pray enough their parent may be healed. Children may take the failure of their strategies as a sign of their own failure.

"I remember for a while after I was diagnosed with M.S., Sean was always saying 'I'm sorry' whenever I was cross at him," recalls his mother, Sharon. "That was definitely not like him. He used to take my reprimands in stride. Now he seemed quite upset at any misconduct and became very anxious about his schoolwork.

"One time he seemed unusually disturbed by a 'B' he got for a report. When I asked him why he made such a big deal out of what was a good effort, he broke into tears. Sean said he didn't want to upset me anymore by doing badly in school. He thought if I wasn't upset at him, maybe I could get better quicker.

"I explained to him," Sharon relates, "that my M.S. had nothing to do with how he did in school or behaved at home. I said that sometimes it seemed to get better and other times I felt worse. What made me feel best of all, however, was my love for him. I let him know it was okay if sometimes he felt sad or angry, he didn't always have to be happy—and that his doing things I sometimes got upset about gave me an opportunity to be a mother. If he had stopped being a rascal, I probably would have become more ill from boredom. Thank God for kids!"

Children may also fear that multiple sclerosis is fatal, contagious, or inherited. They may wonder whether a parent will enter or return to the hospital. They may be reluctant to ask their parents for help or to participate in school activities. They may be unsure of what their parent's limits are or how to ask about them. They may not know what to tell friends or what they can do to help their parent.

Todd is a twelve-year-old boy whose father, Jack, was diagnosed with M.S. when Todd was eight. "It was scary," Todd remembers. "My father would trip sometimes or he would tell me he couldn't play catch because he was tired. But then I'd see him talking to my mom and she would look pretty worried and then he'd go upstairs and lie down. My mom would tell me and my brother to quiet down because my dad wasn't feeling well.

"Well, I thought maybe he was having heart attacks or cancer or something because I was only eight and those were the bad illnesses I had heard about. My grandfather had died when I was six and I remember him going to lie down a lot so I thought maybe my dad was dying. Then one day I came home from school and my aunt was there and she said my mother was with my father at the hospital. I was really scared. When my mother came home for supper she said Dad would be in the hospital for a few days but he'd be okay. Well, the few days seemed incredibly long—I found out later it was ten days—and when he did return he was in a wheelchair.

"Now my parents tell me that they didn't want to worry me by visiting the hospital or telling me what was happening," Todd continues. "But they don't realize how shocked I was to see my dad in a wheelchair all of a sudden. I felt like the floor had disappeared and I was falling through space. I got this horrible feeling in my stomach and I still get it every now and then. I feel like I'm not sure I can trust anyone anymore. When they say my dad will be okay, can I be sure? My parents still don't tell me everything about my dad's M.S. and I feel like I shouldn't be asking too many questions.

"Sometimes my dad and I play in the house," Todd explains. "I push him in his wheelchair and I jump on the back and we whip around. We even knock things over sometimes. We call it roughhousing. We love it. But when my mom catches us doing it she gets really angry with me. She says my dad's sick and I could get him too excited and then he would be worse. My dad says it's not true, but I don't know who to believe and I would rather not hurt my dad than have fun with him, so we don't roughhouse as much as we used to.

"Also, sometimes I'll ask my dad if he wants to go to one of my games or school meetings and he says he'd love to. But my mom often says that it'll tire him out so I shouldn't ask him. I think she feels bad about people seeing him in his wheelchair. We don't ask too many questions in my family, and the M.S. especially is something we don't talk too much about, so I don't know what the real answer is. I feel left out a lot from helping with my dad. My mom tells me not to bring friends home too often so Dad won't feel uncomfortable with strangers around, but I think it's her who really feels bad. I wish I knew the real story," Todd pleads.

These and other concerns can usually be addressed in a simple, straightforward, and comforting style. How a parent responds to a child's concerns is greatly influenced by a parent's or family's own ease of adjustment to the disease. A booklet we highly recommend to parents and children in answering some basic questions about M.S. and as a starting point for discussion is "Someone You Know Has Multiple Sclerosis," published by the Massachusetts Chapter of the National Multiple Sclerosis Society. Write to them at: 400-1 Totten Pond Road, Waltham, MA 02154.

Adjusting to chronic illness in a family is a great challenge and opportunity. The stresses individual family members and the system as a whole undergo may be enormous. But families endure and learn from their experience to better cope with subsequent crises. People may "rise to the occasion" in ways unanticipated by them. Just as weddings and births provide the moment to make vows, calamities and trials present the time to fulfill them. And the immediate family may evolve beyond itself to include within its boundaries of heart—as well as blood—relatives, in-laws, friends, and community.

Helping others comes naturally to us. Perhaps it is the behavior most characteristic of humans. Both in everyday situations and at times of need, our impulse is to reach out, to offer a hand, to help. Even in war we give comfort to the wounded on our side and, sometimes, provide it for the enemy. Yet our natural capacity for generosity and compassion is underrated and often taken for granted. Still, we, and those with whom we live, want to do what we can. A family is a field in which we can practice this most graceful skill.

❖ 4 ❖

Employment

THE IMPACT OF multiple sclerosis extends beyond the relationship one has with family and friends. It may also have a significant effect on one's work and career. First, some employers and employees may be uncomfortable around someone labeled as having multiple sclerosis. Second, M.S. symptoms may rob one of the very skills necessary for a particular profession. Third, fatigue can take away the energy needed to hold down a full-time job or to function effectively in a high-pressure environment. And, finally, the top rung of the ladder, which was once within easy reach, may now seem insurmountably high or dangerously shaky.

For those people whose identities and life satisfaction are intimately linked to their achievements or status at work, M.S. is a major threat to their psychological well-being. Many individuals, as well, find the companionship and camaraderie of the workplace a necessary ingredient of their lives. Deprived of this opportunity because of disability or fatigue, the M.S. person may easily become despondent.

"When I learned that I had M.S.," says Dick, who was a designer in the consumer electronics industry, "I became convinced that it was the end of the line for me at work. I thought I wouldn't be able to keep up with what was expected of me in terms of job perform-ance and in the relationships around the office that were important for career advancement. How could I have lunch with the other guys if I couldn't keep up with them on the sidewalk?

"I made some rash decisions, which I now regret," he continues. "I was confused and angry about my diagno-sis. I was not thinking at all of what I wanted for myself and my family. Instead, I was focused on what I wanted to avoid: doing my job poorly, getting sympathy from my colleagues, giving excuses to my boss. So I quit and we moved out of the city. My talents in design have not been used since. And that's a pity."

Although Dick's frustration and fears are understand-able, there are alternatives to taking action on the basis of conflict and anxiety. It is possible, through setting priorities and creative problem solving, to continue to find enjoyment and meaning through work.

Larry, for example, took his M.S. diagnosis as an opportunity to reflect carefully upon the meaning his life and work had for him. "I was a lawyer who specialized in divorce law. I did my work well and was highly respected by my colleagues and clients. But I really valued mar-riage and family life and I often felt as if I arrived too late in a person's life. I was practicing surgery instead of preventive medicine. And the I-win-you-lose part of the legal process of divorce and settlement never sat well with me. However, I got paid a hell of a lot.

"Once I dealt with the initial impact of finding out I had multiple sclerosis and realized I might have to cut down on some of the sixty- and eighty-hour weeks I was regularly putting in, I actually breathed a sigh of relief. If I'm going to be less 'high powered,' I thought, why not do more of what I wanted. Once I started thinking in those terms, it was an easy step to where I am now.

Larry now practices family law and assists couples with adoption and divorce mediation, helping couples settle their differences as amicably and fairly as possible before entering court. He also counsels law students and their spouses about the trade-offs involved in choosing careers in corporate law, for example, or a public service practice. Despite his illness, he has never been happier.

Some work-related issues are problems to be overcome, some are challenges to transcend illness, and some provide opportunities to transform a person's self-image and develop new resources and skills. The benefits that come from good work well done are too important to be abandoned when illness may threaten the usual ways that those rewards are gained.

It is often the case, however, that what a person does about his employment after being diagnosed is influenced by the response of the people with whom he works. One's colleagues or managers may be viewed as either additional obstacles or available resources to help a person with multiple sclerosis cope with his or her illness.

"I was quite nervous about going back to work after my most recent exacerbation landed me in a wheelchair," reports Paula. "Everyone who knew I had M.S. had been quite supportive after my original diagnosis, but since there had been little change for such a long time the

M.S. was just something that disappeared from everyone's mind.

"Going back to work, I'd have to deal with everybody's questions, no matter how well intentioned. I also knew that people would be wondering whether I'd 'measure up' to the work load. My job is a very high-pressure one to begin with, a lot of people get stressed out; I had my own doubts about whether or not I'd be able to perform at my previous level. My company has terrific disability benefits and I was tempted to try to make a case for my need to stay at home for a longer time.

"But I knew, for me," admits Paula, "that that would only be a way of avoiding my eventual coming to terms with the effect of my M.S. on my work situation. I don't see it as a career buster, but it sure put me on the slow track. I still wonder how much of that is due to my holding back for fear of putting myself under more public scrutiny or the lowered expectations of my managers. I've found it difficult to sit down and talk with them about it. I feel as if I'd be asking for sympathy or special treatment. That's something I have to work out with myself, then I'll deal with my managers."

An employer or manager typically has a complex range of reactions to the diagnosis of M.S. for an employee. She feels concern for the well-being of the employee, has her own personal psychological attitudes about illness, and must consider what an employee's illness or disability means for the organization. A manager is subject to multiple obligations and often may feel constrained as to the amount and kind of support she may give.

Some, of course, are immediately sympathetic and helpful. "The first thing my manager asked me was to tell him about multiple sclerosis and what it meant for me and my family," relates Suzanne. "He wanted to know if there was anything he could do for me. He offered me time off or more flexible hours. Not once in that initial meeting did he express concern as to how my illness could affect him or the company. He was totally focused on my needs. He stepped right out of his typical manager role and became the friend I needed."

Not everyone is as fortunate as Suzanne. As Bill describes, "I was very hesitant to tell my boss that I had M.S. and might need to sit down and rest occasionally or take a few more days off. When I used the words 'multiple sclerosis' he got very anxious and started asking me if there was anyone I thought I could train to take my place. I tried to explain about my illness, but I could see he was just not listening. He made it very clear that there was no place for a 'sick' person in his group. If I couldn't do the job the way he wanted, well. . . ."

The question of whether and what to tell one's employer, manager, or colleagues may be crucial. Even when a manager is sympathetic in a personal way, a worker with M.S. may fear that he will receive less important assignments or fewer and less frequent promotions. On the other hand, if one does not disclose a chronic illness, requests for personal days, sick leave, occasional part-time work, or less travel are unlikely to be granted. We think it is better to be honest more often than not. There are situations, however, where full disclosure is risky, and one is better off saying nothing unless circumstances demand it.

Whatever you do, it is useful to recognize the situation your manager is in. As sympathetic as he may be, what he can do is limited by company policy and by the fact that you are not his sole employee. He may believe that granting you what he views are special favors, such as a modified schedule or more frequent rest periods, may be unfair to the others whom he manages.

Gabe, the manager of a small technical writing group in a high-tech company, felt trapped. "An employee of mine, Sue, has recently been diagnosed with multiple sclerosis. Her double vision and tremors make it difficult for her to do her job in a timely manner. She has to spend a great deal of time at a computer terminal and she just can't be as productive as we need.

"We care a lot about our people here," Gabe points out, "and I offered to help Sue find a new position with the company at the same salary and same level, but she refused. She likes our group and facility a lot and she feels she can't take another loss and adjustment as she's had to do with her illness. However, I can't put my other people in the position where they have to do more work to pick up for Sue.

"I really don't know what to do. I don't want to be in the position where I have to make the decision for Sue to do what's best for the group. I also question whether she'll be happy operating at less than 100 percent for this group when she'd be able to be as productive as she ever was in some other situation more suited to her current physical needs. I'm arranging a meeting with Sue, myself, and our personnel people to try to resolve this situation in as positive a way as possible. I don't think it's her M.S. that's getting in the way here. I think it's Sue's attitude toward her situation. I can empathize with her on a personal level, but I also have responsibilities toward my work."

The attitudes that your employer and your colleagues have about illness will influence their responses to you. Little-known diseases such as multiple sclerosis may generate unconscious fears of contagion. Others will be anxious about how to respond appropriately to a person with a chronic illness. They are also unsure whether they will see physical changes, embarrassing behavior or decline, and disability. Colleagues may be uncomfortable in a role they see more fitting for family and close friends. They may be concerned that working with an ill person may create necessary intimacies they may prefer to avoid.

"I feel bad for Sue," reports Grace, one of her co-workers. "Something like M.S. is a terrible thing to happen to anyone, especially someone like Sue whom we all like so much. But I think she should be trying to get some help from her family or a counselor to help her cope with it. Almost every day she tells me her current condition, how she's feeling, asking me medical questions that I certainly have no idea how to answer, or asking for advice.

"She's less able to do her job and so she avoids it by focusing on her illness. But that just makes it harder for us to do our jobs and she becomes even less productive. She feels as if we're all one family; she hates the idea of being assigned to another group where she could do better work but where we couldn't be as close as she would like. She doesn't fully understand that we are co-workers, not family. We don't even see each other outside work very much. I think Sue's using her belief in our closeness as a way of avoiding her own problems and the lack of support in her life outside of here."

It is important for a person with a chronic illness to recognize the psychological defenses others may employ in an attempt to ward off disease, disability, and, potentially, death. Jacqueline, for example, had a colleague who refused to acknowledge her illness. "If I was out a day or two, she'd ask me where I'd been. If I told her that

I had multiple sclerosis and was very fatigued, she would simply say, 'You're not sick. You look fine to me.' She was convinced I was taking time off to either have an affair or go shopping. Finally, it was just easier to say I had a cold, and leave it at that. It seemed to satisfy her."

Most colleagues express support and want to help. But it may be necessary to educate them about multiple sclerosis, about how it is not contagious, and that the various symptoms may come and go. "The people who worked with me were terrific," reports Suzanne. "They were very upset when I told them my diagnosis, but I noticed some reluctance on their part to ask for more details and some shying away from lunching with me as before. I confided my concern to my best friend at the office and she told me people thought that talking with me about the M.S. would upset me. Now I know they were expressing their own anxieties about the illness by not wanting to talk about it.

"So I took the bull by the horns. I asked everyone to meet with me for a half hour one morning and told them it was a session of 'everything you always wanted to know about M.S. but were afraid to ask.' Everyone came. Several asked if M.S. could be transmitted. Some were shocked that I had a serious illness because I continued to look so well.

"When we finished, a colleague asked me to keep him up to date on my work so he could pitch in if I ever had to be out more than a few days. He didn't want me turning down responsibilities and assignments because I feared I might not be able to complete them. Most sympathetic were the parents who worked and knew what it was like to have conflicting demands on time and attention. From then on, they knew when I could use lunch companions or a telephone call at home when I was resting."

The loss or threatened loss of one's employment can have devastating consequences for both an individual and his or her family. Economic uncertainty and financial hardship, changes in roles and status within the family, and issues of self-image and self-esteem are all affected in major ways by a diagnosis of multiple sclerosis.

The availability of disability insurance, prior savings, company pension plans, and the kinds and amounts of financial resources a family has influence the anxiety with which one faces threats to employment. Another fact that can ameliorate or exacerbate the blow of career instability or change is whether a spouse is or is not currently working. Of course, the situation is made even more difficult by the occasional or anticipated need, or wish, of the spouse to be more available to care for the partner with M.S.

In these kinds of circumstances, the attempt to solve one problem—a spouse getting a job—can intensify another—the person with M.S. feels inadequate because of his or her inability to maintain a full-time position. The pileup of individual stressors creates another and greater kind of stress: an overwhelming sense of defeat and hopelessness. Occasional feelings of this kind are normal. A persistent inability to function without this pervading air of futility is a sign to seek professional counseling and help.

When Sandy became ill from M.S., for example, she had to reduce her working hours. "The result was that my husband, Bill, had to change his job in order to make up for the loss of family income. Bill's new job required greater commuting, which meant he was less available to help me care for our children and cook and clean. I became even more tired, and due to the loss of income we weren't able to hire anybody to help out at home.

"Bill became so exhausted from commuting he was less able to be emotionally supportive of me as I was less able to be for him. The children felt the drop in our energy and time. They became cranky at home and we gave their schoolwork less attention so they also suffered. It seemed we were rolling downhill on an avalanche of troubles."

Sandy continues, "I offered to return to work full-time, but Bill would have none of that. He figured the financial lift would not be worth the trade-off in my fatigue and the taking of even more time away from the children. I just wanted to quit. My M.S. interfered with my ability to get around the house; I had never been so tired in my life, Bill and the kids were suffering terribly. Whatever I touched turned to lead. I felt hopeless. I thought the people I loved would be better off if I were to die.

"Fortunately, I scared myself with my thinking. I had never before considered suicide. I was normally a very happy person, even after my diagnosis. I blurted out how badly I was feeling to my closest friend. She was very sympathetic. She told me she had once felt as terrible as I did and she had gone to a therapist who had been of tremendous help to her. My friend helped me realize that my despair was unique to someone who was ill, but that many people feel overwhelmed by what is currently happening in their lives. I took her advice and saw her therapist, who has been very good for me.

"Bill and I are adjusting better to the many changes we went through in a short period of time. We're establishing routines and not insisting that we live our lives as we had before my illness. Meals are not as lavish, floors are not as clean, and we spend less money on entertainment than before. In some ways our lives are simpler. In some ways, indeed, our lives are better. I suppose we had to go through our rocky period to get to the point where we could see that."

There is much that can be done to prepare yourself and your family to meet the challenges M.S. presents to career plans and life goals. Planning, preparation, and flexibility are key. After receiving a diagnosis, perhaps the best advice is to do nothing. Take a deep breath. Relax. Career and employment changes due to one's choice as well as events beyond one's control are certainly not unusual. If a person approaches the whole issue as an opportunity for career and life-style evaluation, rather than as a crisis-laden reaction to a medical catastrophe, the results are likely to be more satisfying and the process of arriving at them less stressful.

"After my first exacerbation, which pulled me out of work for three weeks," David says, "I became quite anxious. I started searching the want ads for almost any kind of position that would give me some income with flexible hours. I felt as if I needed to make changes right away, before anything else happened.

"I pushed Julie [David's wife], who had been home with our children, to decide what her career was going to be and find an entry-level position somewhere or go back to school part-time. Naturally, the more I pushed the more she resisted. I accused her of being afraid, unsupportive. I was in a real panic. I acted as if the entire future we had imagined together was going to be lost and it was my fault. I had to drive us to create a new future, whether it was what we wanted or not. I felt out of control."

Fortunately, David had a friend, Ben, who had been laid off three years before and had made an extremely successful career adjustment. Ben told David that he and his wife, Elizabeth, had sat down right after his lay-off and decided: (1) the layoff was not Ben's fault and *was not* his responsibility, and (2) creating a new career and life was an opportunity for growth and *was* their respon-sibility. Ben pointed out that David's frantic efforts were a reaction to his feelings of powerlessness rather than a positive response to the new possibilities that were in front of him.

"Ben was of immeasurable help," David remembers. "After that talk with him, I shifted my orientation toward my illness. I began to see it less as some awful thing that happened to me and my family and more as a catalyst for choices and changes that could be very productive for us all."

David and Julie began to give up the belief that they were entitled to get everything they wanted in life quickly and easily, and that they should never get what they didn't want. Their life until M.S. had been like the first love of a marriage. The M.S. precipitated feelings of anger, disillusionment, and despair. "After David's talk with Ben, our optimistic, romantic outlook was tem-pered by a new realism," Julie admits. "Our despair was replaced by hope and faith in ourselves."

David and Julie had long discussions about what was most important to them in their lives and what they truly valued, both as individuals, as a couple, and as a family. David had been on the fast track at work and it had left him little time to spend with his family. An exacerba-tion for him was equivalent to a derailment, and the effort it took David to recoup from his lost time could result in greater fatigue and more frequent or intense symptoms.

It emerged that their bottom-line value was family. It was the anchor around which their other commitments were made. Setting that priority helped other concerns fall more easily into place. David's health, of course, was important, as was Julie's ability to earn money if David's financial position was threatened.

Gradually, decisions were made and a plan emerged. Julie would return to school on a part-time basis to get her degree in a field she wanted to work in; David would begin to explore other positions in his own and other companies that were financially less remunerative but also less demanding and more flexible in time and responsibilities. They anticipated that their combined incomes would be only a little higher than David's former one, but they would have substantially more opportunities to be with and help out each other and their children.

Of course, single parents with multiple sclerosis, especially those with young children, face particularly hard and difficult circumstances. They are less likely to have financial resources, other people in the family who can earn money, useful skills for the job market, or time to develop and obtain new ones. A major source of emotional and material support can be family and friends. Single parents with multiple sclerosis, and statistics show they are overwhelmingly female, may find help from the women's job placement centers and networks that have developed in many areas. Local M.S. societies may also be useful in identifying work opportunities.

Mary had suffered a depression while Erroll was a law student. He had decided to attend school as part of a full-time class during the evening session. "As a result," Erroll explains, "I spent all of my free time studying, leaving little time to spend with Mary and the boys. In fact, until William was four, he hardly knew me. I went from work to school to studying seven days a week."

"So I was relegated to the background," Mary adds, "taking care of house and hearth—forever keeping the children quiet so 'Daddy can work on his books.'" She marvels in retrospect, "How different life became from my fantasy of what a wife and mother's role would be while I was working for the newspaper. It certainly was not all it was supposed to be. What a letdown."

Mary further describes her symptoms. "I had trouble eating and sleeping; I wasn't interested in things and, most of all, I didn't feel like doing anything social, even with my old friends. I felt I had nothing to contribute to the conversation."

"We finally felt as if we had conquered this problem after a combination of couples' therapy and medication," Erroll explains. "I was so relieved that after a difficult year and a half Mary was finally becoming more like herself."

Life then appeared to settle down for this couple who felt they had "paid their dues" and had earned the right to some uncomplicated happiness. Two years later, however, Mary began to feel inordinately fatigued. "Oh, how disappointed I was to see these symptoms return," Erroll volunteers with a frown. "I found myself losing patience with her and with her complaints. I was too busy at work to deal with these problems when I came home to relax."

Mary picks up the story at this point. "This time my eyes became blurry and I seemed to have difficulty moving my stiff legs. I was embarrassed to tell Erroll or anyone about these symptoms for a long time. When I did, he would explode with anger. I also felt it was 'all my fault.' I began to feel worse about myself each day.

"Finally," Mary continues with a pained expression, "one day I fell while walking upstairs, and I decided it was time to talk to our family doctor about how I was feeling, no matter how Erroll reacted." Mary then underwent diagnostic testing and was referred to a psychiatrist because of her previous history of depression. This gentleman was quite perceptive and immediately referred her to a neurologist. "Of course, the diagnosis took many months, and many arguments with Erroll erupted in the meantime."

By the time Mary received her diagnosis of multiple sclerosis, Erroll had been angry and resentful most of their time together. He describes them at that point as having "multiple problems, too numerous to solve." They had become so far apart that they decided to separate almost immediately.

Mary describes the first few weeks of living as a single parent as "relief time. I was my own person again, beholden to no one for whatever time I needed to rest. Then reality set in," she explains, "and I realized I would need a job to support the three of us as well as restore my much damaged ego.

"It was my supportive next door neighbor, Joan, who had been following our saga over the past year with real empathy, and who had suggested I contact the local M.S. Society with ideas for job placement," Mary explains. "Though they had no definitive listings to give me, the gentleman in the Patient Services sector of the Society was exceedingly helpful. He spent hours with me on the phone that week and was so patient (despite being a man) that I realized Erroll was just too insensitive to deal with—and not representative of his gender at all. All what had happened between us was not only my fault."

The M.S. Society had a single-parent group for newly diagnosed M.S. persons that was to begin the next week. Though it involved some transportation and baby-sitting arrangements, Mary organized coverage to attend. She felt supported and validated for the first time that year as people listened empathetically to her story and made some practical suggestions for her future.

Mary's work experience had been in soliciting advertisements for the city newspaper. She had been effective in her job for several years prior to marriage and left work only as Erroll felt threatened by her sharing her time and loyalties with others. Now, however, she found herself hesitant to reenter the world of work. "I wondered," she explains, "whether I should share the truth about my illness with a potential employer. Would anyone be flexible enough to understand my fatigue and any possible attacks that may hinder my productivity?" Mary felt that she needed the companionship as well as the economical support from the marketplace, but because of Erroll's rejection of her and the complications of the disease, she was frightened to try.

She seriously considered her potential as an employee, and together with her support group of other M.S. persons, Mary came to believe once again in her capabilities. "A friend recommended that I apply to the corporation in our town that has been known to support the handicapped," she says. "In that way, they would automatically be kind to me when I needed assistance." Mary was excited with their response. The company published a weekly communication journal and required advertisements from local merchants to defray the costs. "I was perfect for the job," Mary exudes. "I did not require any training, and could arrange my own weekly schedule as long as the work was completed.

"Without the benefit of networking with others who have been in my scary position, I would never have regained my self-esteem," Mary admits. "Friends have commented on my mood changes in the past several months, and I just chuckle. I was lucky to have the assistance of good friends in adjusting to my disease and my divorce. I hope other single parents will be as fortunate as I."

Most important, however, at times of stress and adjustment to disease, it is essential to refrain from serious decision making concerning employment changes. Remissions can occur and a job can again become manageable. Retraining and rethinking of employment decisions take time and serious rational planning, and the number of enlightened employers who are more flexible in assigning responsibilities to all chronic disease persons is increasing each year due to governmental restrictions. Equal opportunity employment is certainly more prevalent as a deserved right than ever before.

✦ 5 ✦

But You Look So Well, Dear

AN OVERWHELMING SENSE of fatigue is one of the most familiar and discouraging symptoms of multiple sclerosis. It may be caused by such factors as muscle weakness, spasticity, incoordination of gait, anxiety, depression, fever from infection, or rise in body temperature from hot weather. It saps your strength to do the simplest of daily chores. These attacks of fatigue may last several minutes or hours to days or weeks at a time, and all a person can do at such times is rest.

The "fatigue factor" is so debilitating that the sufferer easily loses the will to fight it. Louise, the psychiatrist, was highly motivated to continue her life as normally as she could despite her M.S. Some days she would walk without aid, other days she would use a cane. "I would never let my difficulty in getting around keep me from doing errands, lunching with colleagues, or seeing patients," she says. "I was quite proud of myself, really; I thought I was demonstrating how 'one must go on' despite hardship and difficulties.

88

"But when the fatigue came," Louise continues, "all my good intentions went out the door. I just wanted to sit. I didn't want to see people. I felt as if I were encased in a suit of twelfth-century armor. I didn't even have the energy to think. That was probably the worse part. All I could do was pray for that great weight of fatigue to leave."

Often, M.S. persons complain that they feel particularly fatigued in the summer, when the weather is most humid. For these people, sunbathing and beaching cease to be comfortable pastimes. Even commuting to work on the bus or subway can be taxing during the hottest times of the year. Louise describes how difficult it was for her to keep a lecture date during the summer when her air-conditioned car was being repaired. "I glibly told the chairman of the function that I could easily take the subway from my office to the university," she explains, "but by the time I arrived at the lecture hall, I could hardly stand. I explained that I would need some rest time along with a pitcher of cold water. Finally, I adjusted to the air-conditioning and could begin my talk."

Because Louise was both relieved at her improvement and puzzled by her increased fatigue, she discussed this incident with her neurologist. She was fearful that a new attack was beginning. "After your last exacerbation, you were probably left with some abnormal areas where the myelin was lost," he patiently explained, "and the hot weather decreases the clarity of the messages from your brain not due to a new attack, but because of the residue from the old one."

Fatigue accounts for a large percentage of the frustration of those with M.S. who may not be wheelchair-bound. Others assume that if one looks well or moves well, one *is* well. People, even loved ones, have difficulty understanding what the fatigue factor consists of, why the person with M.S. wakes up as tired as he or she went to sleep, or why the afternoon hours may be the most trying.

The fatigue factor is one of the most frustrating symptoms of multiple sclerosis because the cause, not its effects, is invisible to others. How you look may also be incongruent with how you feel. Marilyn's experience illustrates both of these factors.

"I was a model working for a well-known agency when I first came for help. I had M.S. but something else seemed terribly wrong. I had a sense of not knowing who I was, of not being who I seemed. I was tired all the time and depressed. I had lots of skill and taste in clothes and makeup, but my exhaustion was undermining my best efforts to look good."

Marilyn had particular problems with her father and older brother, Tom, who were her sole support system. When she complained of fatigue to her father, he would chuckle and give her money for a new blouse or coat. In order to please him, she would often wear his latest gift the next time they met. "She's thirty-one and still my spoiled girl," he would respond.

Her older brother, who had more family responsibilities, would listen to this exchange and shrug his shoulders. He was frustrated with his sister for "her manipulative ways of dealing with our father."

Marilyn's father was a seventy-four-year-old gentleman who knew his daughter's diagnosis, but had not yet emotionally accepted it. He was both proud of her vibrant, successful appearance as well as concerned about his own aging and mortality. He attempted to deny the great anxiety her illness created in him by reinforcing his image of her youth and beauty. He would interrupt her complaints of fatigue with "but you look so well, dear."

Her father's compliments frustrated Marilyn. She made a striking appearance, but how she felt did not blend with how she appeared. Each of us has a sense of ourselves different from the way others see us; for the person with multiple sclerosis, this may be even truer and more confusing.

Some family members may perceive the person with M.S. as lazy or spoiled when, as in Marilyn's case, weakness and fatigue are the only symptoms present. It is important, therefore, to share information as well as emotions with the important person in one's life in order to overcome the tendency toward denial and relieve the feelings of aloneness. If no one is available to share or understand these feelings, as was the case with Marilyn despite her father's concern, then anxiety and depression increase.

Although it was important for Marilyn to continue to feel good about her appearance, it also became essential for her to share the less superficial aspects of her life with her father and brother. Marilyn's family could have given her more useful support if she had frankly discussed her symptoms and her need to rest.

Not all parents, however, are free enough of their own psychological concerns to be as helpful as possible. Anger, depression, and fearfulness as well as denial are common responses. Some parents, such as Marilyn's father, dread the possibility of illness, advanced age, or dependency on others. They find it difficult to extend themselves. Family members could ease a lot of the painful feelings and unnecessary deception if they communicated openly about the sources of their feelings.

Fatigue can often be confused with depression. The fatigue factor we are describing is not a depression, although everyone is made unhappy by a disease that interrupts life's routine or disrupts plans. While one eats and sleeps normally and continues to enjoy activities and finds enjoyment with one's relatives and friends, there will have to be some changes made in how and when interests are pursued; time has to be put aside for rest.

Marilyn's frustration and feelings of depression were not due solely to her disease; she also felt a strong need to cover up her fatigue, to keep her family and herself from acknowledging it. Her intense negative thinking surprised not only her family but herself as well. Her perceptions and goals about life became distorted. She questioned her work, her present, and her future and found it increasingly more difficult to vent these questions or change her mood.

Barbara is a young housewife whose husband, an efficiency expert for a local company, is in the habit of leaving her lists of what to accomplish each day. She is so minimally disabled by her M.S. that both she and her husband are comfortable in denying her symptoms in actual conversation with each other. On the days that she is particularly fatigued, however, she feels intensely guilty at her failure to carry out her list.

One morning, her listed tasks for the day were carrying the wood from the cellar and shoveling the snow from her walk. She struggled with these all morning. By lunchtime, her thoughts became negative and pessimistic.

"I felt like the goldfish in my kitchen fishbowl," admits Barbara, "trapped and unable to do anything on my own. I had so much self-doubt, I couldn't accomplish, or even attempt, anything for days afterward."

Barbara's blues were the result of her own distorted thinking. "I believed that if I couldn't finish the chores on my husband's list, that I was good for nothing. I saw myself as caged, stupid, and powerless."

In such moods, Barbara felt like a failure for having her disease. She was guilty and disappointed with herself. She was irritated with and lost interest in the people around her. She became incapable of making any decisions. Although her depressing thoughts were not accurate, Barbara believed them to be true. A self-defeating cycle of negative thoughts and inaction was established.

"I would return home from work every day," Glen, Barbara's husband, says. "Barbara, who's usually nicely made-up and enthusiastic, would just sit there, not moving. When she was in one of her down moods, Barbara seemed to dislike herself, me, the kids— everyone and everything. It was frightening. I couldn't talk to her and I didn't know what to do. Sometimes I'd try to tease her out of her blues. Other times I'd lecture or shout. Nothing worked."

Glen also felt powerless to do anything to help Barbara at home. He could not consider leaving his job, which had excellent medical benefits. "Also, to be honest about it, I didn't want to be closer to home. I needed the whole hour of my commute to calm down from work and be able to face 'Barbara's Blues.' Some days I had to force myself to return home. I used to fantasize about driving past my exit on the expressway and just keep moving on."

In Barbara and Glen's case, their anger and depression were the result of not adequately adjusting to her multiple sclerosis and fatigue coupled with marital conflicts that had begun to emerge. In addition to addressing those latter issues, however, Barbara needed to feel less overwhelmed by her fatigue.

Barbara and Glen benefited from counseling to help her identify the thoughts that predated her paralyzing negativity. Glen needed help to examine his unrealistic and demanding expectations. When Barbara no longer felt that she had to accomplish Glen's objectives, she started to take small steps toward attaining what she wanted and could manage each day. A benevolent circle of positive thinking and successful action was initiated. Both her depression and his anger lessened.

Even when not exacerbated by depression, fatigue can be disabling as it affects the stamina and the energy needed to accomplish everyday tasks. Adjusting to fatigue becomes easier when one sets priorities. A person's ebb and flow of family involvement and activity becomes "normal."

When June was diagnosed with multiple sclerosis four years ago, her two sons, ages six and five, were told by their father only that their mother had to lie down on the couch frequently to keep the furniture from moving. At these times, they'd been told, they had to play quietly with their toys. June needed to rest two or three times each afternoon for as long as half an hour.

When the boys asked what would happen if Mom didn't lie down, their father had to stop and think about how to respond appropriately to their need for information. In the best tradition of a clever parent, he asked them a question, "What do *you* think would happen if Mom didn't lie on the couch?" "It would fly away," they both responded gleefully. This levitation theory gained acceptance in the household as did Mom's fatigue. Everyone's stress and anxiety was reduced by good humor and mutual support.

It is difficult, however, for many people with M.S. to set priorities and limits for daily behavior because of their high expectations for themselves. They do not want to compromise their ambitions and goals, and in fact, this need not be the case. What is required is not so much reducing what one wants as it is changing the time and style expected to attain it. Trying too hard, needing to please others, and living life in a driven manner leads to anxiety, fatigue, and, inevitably, depression. This is particularly so for those whose reservoir of energy is limited to begin with.

Fran had been the recognized family caretaker for many years. Prior to her parents' death, all of her siblings agreed that she was the one who would care for them in her home. Others in the family visited on a weekly basis, but it was always Fran who ran things day to day. She would do all the errands, take them for doctors' visits and on outings, and be there to cheer up these two souls who had been weakened by both their heart ailments and fear of aging. Because she was the only one of four children not to marry, Fran was considered the "least busy" of the family. That she was regularly employed by the Visiting Nurse Association in their area added to the family's view that she was the most suited for this task. As Fran's brother would explain, "Surely she was more appropriate to help with the elderly through both her training and her profession than we, who were accountants, businessmen, and flight attendants." Further, she had no children of her own. They believed as did she, that life would be lonely without her parents present.

After several years as family caretaker, Fran finally found herself living alone. Her parents had died in the past two years, and after all of the possessions and legalities had been taken care of, she was at last in a position to plan for her own free time. At her forty-fifth birthday, the family gathered to "toast her" good-heartedly and questioned how she would now "fill her time." Each family member had a recommendation as to how she would now be able to further assist them all. Baby-sitting, errand running, housesitting—tasks that were designed to make all of their lives easier—were explored. Fran laughed with the group, but was honestly taken aback by their apparent though subtle insistence that she continue to spend all of her free time in family service.

What Fran did not mention to her family that evening was that she had been feeling poorly lately. She had seen her family doctor just that week, complaining of what she had considered "strange symptoms." She had been feeling somewhat dizzy, and the vertigo she experienced made it difficult for her to drive. Because her job involved climbing flights of stairs several times a day to visit patients, she was aware of a stiffness and fatigue in her legs. Her physician, an old family friend, listened kindly to Fran's complaints and explained to her that these symptoms were not unusual ones to experience after stressful times. She had been so busy caring for her parents, and then their possessions, that he recommended she take some time off from work.

Fran rested for a full week. Her symptoms seemed to disappear, and she returned to work. Several months later, however, the stiffness in her legs reappeared. This time, as she arose in the morning from a full night's sleep, she was more aware of having to move around to relax her legs. She also felt more fatigued throughout the day, but especially in the evening, than she could ever remember. Of course, when she mentioned this to her sister, the reply was, "But Fran, you've never looked better—and you should, with all of this free time." Because Fran's family never adjusted to her refusal to make their lives easier, her siblings would eye her strangely whenever she complained about her own health. She soon learned to keep silent.

Six months later, Fran decided to visit a neurologist with whom she was associated through the VNA. After giving her a spinal tap, numerous other diagnostic tests, and listening to her medical history he finally labeled her symptoms as other than psychological adjustments to her aloneness. After he gave her the diagnosis of M.S., he explained that some of life's more painful experiences can, however, accentuate symptoms that have already existed, though certainly her parents' deaths were not responsible for her disease.

Fran's usually amiable smile fades from her face as she recalls this portion of her history. "As I was certain about my diagnosis," she recalls, "I decided to call a family meeting and present all the facts to my sister, two brothers, and their spouses." Though this was a difficult evening for Fran, she understood, as a health-care professional, that open communication was necessary in order for all of them to adjust to her news. "I told them that I decided not to keep anything from them all, because it was the whole family's problem." At first there was much hesitation and denial in their responses. Fran met these statements head-on. "I am not asking any of you to look after me," she explained, "I merely want you all to respect my setting my own schedule, and my fatigue, despite how I look. You see, I plan to take good care of myself, but I want you all to understand." Fran's strong belief in the value of communication finally touched her family. They soon began to listen to her story with their hearts, perhaps for the first time.

The very next week, as Fran had to refuse an offer to visit her sister in order to celebrate her nephew's birthday, she openly said, "My M.S. is bothering me today. I think I have to take it easy and stay home. Thanks for asking me."

Fran learned a difficult but important lesson as a result of her M.S. She says, "I learned to be a more honest person, and to value and respect myself more. Instead of driving myself to help out whenever I was asked, I began to prioritize my time commitments. This was a different me, and it was hard for my family to adjust. The disease did help"—she smiles in recall—"perhaps it gave me an excuse to do what I should have done years earlier."

Chuck was diagnosed with multiple sclerosis while he was in the middle of an exciting career as a corporate consultant. His profession involved a lot of traveling, working long hours, lunch and dinner meetings, and a need to regularly meet and cultivate new clients. Chuck's family and friends would often compliment him on his ambition and achievements. But even before his recent illness, they were concerned about what seemed to be a frenetic and compulsive drive to succeed.

"Although my M.S. affected my ability to walk," Chuck relates, "I didn't allow it to hold me back. I kept up the same schedule as before. I took taxis more often and would occasionally use a cane, and I even used wheelchairs at airports to save myself from those long cross-terminal walks. I was more careful with my scheduling, but I didn't do any less than before. I was just more tightly structured.

"I gave all my clients as much attention and time as ever. My wife thought I should do more work on the telephone or by computer terminal, but I felt I needed to keep my clients happy with a lot of in-person contact. I guess I assumed that if I wasn't perfect for them all the time they'd let me go.

"Who got shortchanged in the process?" continues Chuck. "My family and my personal interests, of course. I had had little time for them before my illness, but after M.S. struck and I had to do as much as before with less mobility, they were the first to go. I was going like crazy, doing my job, but I began to feel less satisfaction than before. In fact, I felt lonely and even depressed.

"I also noticed that even though my leg wasn't holding me back, I would experience waves of fatigue that I'd. never had before. I could barely keep my eyes open and I was drinking coffee as if it were jet fuel. I needed it in order to keep functioning."

Chuck's wife, Laurel, points out, "I urged Chuck to slow down. I said that although it might seem to him as if his M.S. were limited to how it affected his walking, it really did impact upon him in other ways. He thought he looked so good, but I could see that he wasn't able to keep up the pace he had before. He looked tired. He was fooling himself to think he could go on as before and treat the M.S. as if it weren't there. I knew that we had to reevaluate his business style, and maybe even his business goals.

"Both of us had read about home-based businesses and while theoretically Chuck's office was in our home, he did so much traveling that he actually worked more out of an airplane seat and briefcase. As he realized the cost to him and us, and potentially to his health, of pushing himself in the same way as before, he became more willing to explore other options. We checked out computers and modems and how other consultants managed their businesses."

"Laurel convinced me," Chuck goes on, "to be frank with my clients about my limitations. I was reluctant to do so because I never felt truly confident about myself or my work, which probably explains, at least in part, my need to succeed at almost any cost. To my surprise— and satisfaction—they all indicated that they were, indeed, very pleased with my work and would be happy to accommodate my needs. In fact, they were surprised that I had always done as much traveling as I had done, even before the illness. What they had always wanted was the result. They did not particularly care about how I got the job done.

"Once I was able to pull back on the travel, I found that I had more time to spend with the family and for myself. I would get fatigued as before, sometimes that seemed independent of whatever amount of work I was putting in, but I was more able to take a rest or nap. I also saw that as good as it was, my work had suffered from exhaustion. Of course, I can't say my personality has changed, but I think my life and schedule are more balanced and we're all a lot happier and more at ease."

The stress that may contribute to disease exacerbations can be greatly reduced in realistic and supportive families, like Jane's, where the fatigue factor was openly discussed and adjusted to. The vicious cycle of increased fatigue and stress can be eliminated. The first step in overcoming problems is to admit that they exist, and the hidden dilemma of the fatigue factor—"but you look so well, dear"—needs to be addressed.

Perhaps one of the most discouraging and frightening aspects of multiple sclerosis is the ever-present possibility of an exacerbation, or worsening, of symptoms. No matter how long or briefly one's M.S. has been stable, an attack that leaves the sufferer more impaired than before may occur. Because of this unpredictable element, many people with M.S. are particularly careful to make the best possible use of their "well time," which can create its own kind of subtle pressures and difficulties.

"I noticed some slightly different sensations in my body one day," recalls Jonathan. "My legs felt a little heavier, and once I even had trouble hitting the brake pedal. That really bothered me and I went to bed somewhat anxious. Falling asleep is never easy for me because of the pins and needles I get in my feet, but this night I was more edgy than usual.

"About three A.M. I woke up. I couldn't be sure if my legs were there or not. I tried moving them, but I couldn't tell if they had shifted. My body seemed to be cut off at the waist. I was scared, but, I remember, what I felt most was anger—that I might have to be hospitalized for a short time, taking me away from my work; that I had missed a recent opportunity to travel with my family; that projects might have to be put on hold; and at my damn disease. I wished that I had been more directed with my time, that I had been more driven to get things accomplished. Fortunately, the attack lasted just that night and I had stabilized by morning. Since then, however, I am more unlikely to put things off."

As Jonathan points out, his predominant emotion that frightening night was anger at having wasted time and energy. Because many people fear exacerbation, they react, as Jonathan did, with energy and enthusiasm to their "well time," or period of remission.

Some people with multiple sclerosis seem more impatient when they are in remission. This is partly due to a need to get as much accomplished as possible while there is time. To a person who may be facing a return of symptoms at any moment, down time is time wasted. Also, just as there is more energy available to do what he wants, a person in remission is able to fight and argue more fully. The lifting of fatigue enables the M.S. person to interface with life, in all its aspects, more easily, and the different sides of one's personality become more visible as well. Such a person is motivated to deal with some of life's conflict areas while they have the physical, mental, and emotional resources to do so.

During "well times," people feel more confident and independent. They are more willing to confront those— spouse, friend, employer, parent—upon whom they rely during periods of fatigue, stress, and exacerbation. Remarks Jonathan, "My wife was ambivalent about my 'well periods.' Although she was truly joyous about how good I felt and what I could do, she did not look forward to my overly ambitious projects and my arguing to convince her of them. She felt, and rightly so I think, that many of my ventures and adventures were really attempts to prove something to myself. They were not things I wanted and would enjoy over the long run. I was trying to 'will' myself to health and I'd get annoyed when she raised what were quite sensible objections to my plans."

We see here an understandable tendency by the person with multiple sclerosis to deny the realities of the up-and-down, unpredictable nature of the disease. Although Jonathan had made a good adjustment to his diagnosis and disease, every remission, no matter how brief or mild, gave him hope for a "cure" or permanent stability. Even his employer reaped the benefits and felt the brunt of Jonathan's remission.

On the one hand, Jonathan was excited about taking on new assignments at work. He was highly competent and could manage a heavy load. His employer liked him, respected his abilities, and was sad and disappointed when Jonathan's M.S. was diagnosed. He, as much as anyone, wanted Jonathan to continue to be successful.

On the other hand, both Jonathan and his employer knew that if an exacerbation should occur, Jonathan would simply be unable to deliver what he had agreed to.

Projects would be incomplete and people would be very reluctant to put pressure on Jonathan either to give the assignments to others or to finish them up. The situation would be in a hold period. It seemed to be an insoluble dilemma, and both Jonathan and his employer felt hurt and angry with each other for the position which they were in. Each wanted to do the right thing for himself, the other person, and the company.

Eventually, it was Jonathan's wife, Sheila, a lawyer, who suggested a way out. She proposed that they draw up a "gentlemen's agreement" that would explain the conditions under which Jonathan would hand over responsibility for his projects to another employee while maintaining the opportunity to continue to work on them. It was Jonathan's task to keep specified fellow employees up to date on his work so they could take over if necessary. With goodwill on all sides, the agreement was utilized to everyone's advantage several months later when an exacerbation forced Jonathan to stop working full-time.

The disappointment that Jonathan felt at the time of his exacerbation was tempered somewhat by the realistic way in which he had prepared for it. His agreement with his employer not only helped his career, it also kept the future's unpleasant possibilities and workable alternatives before him.

Not everyone deals with the end of remission as well as Jonathan. Some people feel guilty that they have allowed their long-term "well time" to slip by without having used it to their best advantage. They wish they had that time back. Rather than doing what they can with the time and resources they now have available, they mourn their lost time. Often, this disappointment and regret slips into depression and despair.

Some people may project their guilt onto others and

blame their spouses for not encouraging them to use their "well time" wisely. They may insist that their family obligations forced them to waste their energy on less worthwhile or less interesting pursuits.

"When my most recent exacerbation occurred," observes Jane, "I was unusually irritable with the children and my husband. I asked them why we had wasted so much time watching TV or doing errands, why the children had been playing with friends so often, losing 'quality time' with me, why my husband seemed so concerned with work when he knew how little time we had when I could easily get around.

"It took me a little while before I realized that they had their own lives to live and that part of their adjustment to my M.S. was to live them as normally as possible. My demands for them to adapt so much of their activities to the changes in my illness were unfair, especially because they were so supportive when I needed their help. I got in touch with how much I was denying my anger at my illness, my sadness at being unable to join in some activities, and my despair at the weakening of my strength and mobility."

Jane's reactions are a normal, though unpleasant, response to the loss of well-being that exacerbations bring. With support, understanding, and realism, these reactions tend to be short-lived. It is important to recognize, however, that a person does need to be able to grieve the end of a period of remission.

Remission, exacerbation, "well time," fatigue—all these are important aspects of the multiple sclerosis "experience." To mistake fatigue for laziness, remission for cure, exacerbation for permanence, and "well time" for one's last chance are grave and unnecessary errors. It is more useful to view them as parts of a process of change and adjustment with which individuals and their families, employers, and friends must be aware and cope. The unpredictability of the course or prognosis of multiple sclerosis presents a special challenge to all.

✦ 6 ✦

Process of Adjustment

MULTIPLE SCLEROSIS AFFECTS people in various ways. For some, the disease is relatively "benign" with minor symptoms that do not impact upon one's functioning or do so minimally. For a very few others, it is a terrible scourge, affecting movement, balance, coordination, vision, and the mind in rapid and disheartening succession. Of course, this sort of M.S. presents its own problems of adjustment for family, friends, and patient.

On the other hand, many people have symptoms that progress to a certain level of impairment—use of a cane or a wheelchair, for example—and then remain more or less stable for many months or years until there is a new progression of symptoms and disability. The focus of this chapter is on the problem of adjustment that is most often characteristic of the illness.

The medical literature has described numerous patterns of M.S. Because symptoms differ in each individual, even at the same age, the anxieties experienced by those with M.S. and their loved ones are well founded. As a result, complications in family adjustments vary as do the physical and psychological ramifications of the illness. M.S. symptoms differ in both intensity as well as in frequency; therefore, it may help to classify the four major patterns of M.S.

About 20 percent of the M.S. population experience little to no disability. These persons have a comparatively benign form of the disease. This does not preclude fatigue, anxiety, and family adjustment problems, but it does mean that these people can continue with a normal or near-normal schedule and little interruption in activities of daily living.

Close to 25 percent of M.S. patients have an exacerbating-remitting form, which involves more frequent attacks that clear up—though less completely. These persons can look forward to long periods of stability, but they are often laced with mild disability. Mild to moderate adjustments in life-style and work habits may be advisable during periods of exacerbations.

About 40 percent of those with M.S. experience a chronic-relapsing form. This type is often punctuated by episodic increments. Remissions do occur, but they are less often and with less completeness. These individuals may experience plateaus in the progression of symptoms; but ultimately most experience moderate disabilities in the long run. For these people, work and daily activities should be planned well in advance.

The severest pattern of disability, the chronic-progressive form of M.S., is seen in approximately 15 percent of sufferers. Without the benefit of remission, an insistent and dramatic worsening of old symptoms along with the introduction of new ones leads to increasing loss of functional skills. This smallest group may require assistance in daily living and may have limited opportunities for employment, except by creative planning and strong personal initiative.

Adjusting to multiple sclerosis is particularly challenging because of the peculiar nature of this chronic disease. Just as one thinks that the waters of change are calm, and smooth sailing lies ahead, wham! A boatful of hopes, expectations, goals, and plans is upset, and one feels the desperation of beginning all over again. Neither complete stability nor an inevitable downward progression is typical of M.S. Thus, what one most expects is the unexpected.

An individual with M.S. goes through a back-and-forth process of adjustment and readjustment that accompanies each remission and new exacerbation. Because each new attack can alter the physical, psychological, and social conditions of a person's life, the need to adapt to change itself becomes intensified with this illness. Uncertainty about the future never ends.

An individual with M.S., for example, may interpret minor changes in how one feels as evidence of an exacerbation, and each exacerbation may be considered a first step toward total disability. It is easy to see how the chronic threat of exacerbation can play upon the anxieties of even those who have made successful adjustments to their illness.

"It shakes me up quite a bit," relates Jim, a writer, "when I awaken at two or three or four in the morning unable to feel my legs. I call that time my 'hour of the wolf.' I lie there and try to move them, which it seems I do, but I have difficulty telling. They seem so heavy and at the same time not there, as if I've been cut off at the waist.

"I don't wake my wife because it's probably just a false

alarm, but I feel as if *this is it*. Maybe this is the event that will place me in a wheelchair or leave me less mobile than before. Maybe this morning I'll be unable to walk downstairs or go to work or care for the children. Or maybe these sensations are just transient discomforts, soon to pass, leaving me physically no worse but well reminded of the peculiar nature of this damn disease.

"I try to get my legs over the bed onto the floor and I test them to see if they'll support my weight. They're so stiff. But I get myself up and start walking slowly around the dark room, balancing with one hand touching the wall. As my legs limber up, I go around the house, pleased that I can walk but unsure whether my legs are worse off than before.

"Back in bed, I lie awake thinking about the disease, disability, and death—and cradled in the arms of philosophy I drift off to sleep, often to be awakened two or three other times that night. In the morning, usually no worse than weary, I go about my day. But I feel as if whispers of mortality have been placed in my ear. I hope my awareness of life's fragility enables me to be more compassionate of others."

Some people are not as fortunate as Jim. Exacerbations do occur, and the level of disability slips a notch. Jeffrey's story is such a case. Jeffrey had been an insulin-dependent juvenile diabetic for as long as he could remember. Though his diabetes had been described as a "brittle" case, hard to control even with daily injections, he had adjusted to his fate. He didn't take driving lessons after he turned sixteen, as all his friends did, because of his present though infrequent reactions—he was known to lose consciousness, which could very well affect his ability to maintain control of a car. Nonetheless, his career as an architectural draftsman was well under way. As he describes, "I felt as if statistically I was protected from future disease, as if I had already paid my dues. Life was fairly routine—and not half bad."

But then, suddenly, Jeffrey's hands became tremulous and incoordinate at various times. He refused to believe it to be a permanent situation, and so withheld telling his boss for several weeks. Finally, he could not wait any longer. "I found myself drawing and erasing the same line repeatedly. I needed help to complete my present assignment."

"I advised Jeff to visit his family doc," continues Ed, his boss. "He was a valuable employee, always motivated and cheerful. I never believed that his time with our firm was limited."

Jeffrey was diagnosed as having a chronic-progressive form of M.S. His story is noteworthy. Despite numerous complications resulting from both of his diseases, he has never ceased to search for an enriched way of life. Despite all the threats to him, he and his family have never wavered from appreciating and supporting each other in a positive and constructive manner.

"I had to quit my job, although Ed was disappointed that I made this decision so quickly," Jeff explains. "I could not finish tasks on my own without assistance; I began to question my own skills. It played havoc on my self-esteem."

Jeff's wife, Karen, continues with what she refers to as "our story": "We spent many an evening brainstorming for a good idea. Jeff has always been bright and flexible." He had periods of denial mixed with depression during these times, Karen admits, "but he has never been a depressed personality. He would become aggressively practical at these planning times," she adds, "and then I

would perceive his anxiety, and let him continue."
Reading Jeff's nonverbal communication cues became
an even more important role for Karen during this
difficult period.

"Finally, I believed we had it. The idea seemed so
simple. Jeff would apply to a state rehabilitation commis-
sion for funding to take courses at our local community
college in accounting." The couple rejoiced at their
apparently effective planning. Jeff could use a computer
to solve accounting tasks, and his hand tremors would
not interfere with his problem-solving ability. "I then
hoped I could regain independence," Jeff adds.

The funding was granted, and Jeff began his first
course. Though he did quite well, he was unable to
complete the first semester because of fatigue coupled
with a gradual loss of strength in both legs. After six
months, Jeff became wheelchair-dependent. "I then
found that the school building and the third-floor
classroom were not as wheelchair-accessible as I had
assumed."

"I began to discover the real definition of the word
'progressive,'" Jeff admits. "I was hampered by poorly
coordinated hands, then paralyzed legs, and increasing
fatigue, all of which certainly limited my work potential." Again the couple began brainstorming. Karen
continues, "I had begun a small business of making gift
items for the Christmas season," she explains. "I have
always been fond of arts and crafts, but never before had
the inclination to turn my hobby into a business." With
Jeff home to care for their two young sons, Karen felt
free to develop her talent, and thus became the primary
wage earner.

She noticed that two items sold quite well, and she and
Jeff planned how they could all work together to mass-

produce these gifts. "We began to all sit around the kitchen table and work," Jeff relates. "I soon noticed how close we were all becoming. I was amazed. The feelings were different but so good." Karen, too, was thrilled with the progress of her family. She spent hours during the day visiting local merchants to receive orders, and then would organize Jeff and the boys to contribute by making her unique wreaths. "Business boomed," she notes. "Soon I had to hire more people and convert our garage into a small factory."

"It seemed in those years that just as things were settling down and going well, another jolt would occur," Jeff recalls. "It was time for a diabetic complication to appear." Jeff's left foot became gangrenous, beginning at the toe and continuing up the leg. The surgeon told him the leg required amputation as soon as possible.

As a result of this decision, more adaptive aids became necessary for this brave man and his supportive group. "We needed help at this juncture," Karen describes. The family entered therapy in order to focus on how they all were able to work together in a more original manner, and not necessarily just harder. "I refused to give up," Jeff says. The counselor helped them redefine their goals, and as a result they moved to a neighboring, less costly home that was more wheelchair-accessible and where Jeff could have the benefit of bed rest in a more central area of the house.

The family was continuing its journey in a successful manner. As a group, they continually pledged love and never lost the faith that their commitment to each other was stronger than the discomforts and setbacks they faced. Similarly, as Jeff chooses his medical team carefully, he respects them all, and they all in turn respect him and the way he faces his life. "All who treat him appear to appreciate his courage and gentleness," Karen boasts. "What a man I married!"

At this point, Jeff has had a good couple of years, and his spirits have remained high despite some minor setbacks. One significant symptom occurred that frustrated him more than most others. "Suddenly I developed vertigo or a spinning dizziness that my doctor told me was common but wouldn't last. During these times I was most comfortable in bed, but bored," he admits. Karen picks up on this uncomfortable complication, "We continued to visit the doctor, several times a month, and he tried a variety of new and old medicines, none of which worked. Jeff was tempted to give up then, but the boys and I wouldn't let him."

Finally, their neurologist suggested that Jeff try a transderm scopolamine patch, which delivers an anti-vertigo drug through the skin into the bloodstream, behind his ear. "I couldn't believe how wonderful I felt when these awful feelings cleared," Jeff recalls. The family was jubilant. As predicted, these uncomfortable symptoms disappeared, and the family was again on its way to continued productivity.

Though Jeff's symptoms have continued, the warmth, spirit, and family commitment have continued also. His M.S. has now become more stabilized coincident with every other month, when he receives Cytoxan intravenously over an eight-hour period at a day-care unit of a local hospital. (This treatment followed an initial two-week course of daily Cytoxan as an inpatient.) After each outpatient treatment—he must receive six a year—he can return home. The Cytoxan treatments are part of a study Jeff is participating in. The medication is being administered in accordance with the protocol of the Northeast Cooperative Study Group, a collection of university investigators and M.S. clinics in the northeastern United States. Neither Jeff nor his trusted doctor knows for certain what the long-range benefits or problems will be, but so far Jeff has had his best two years in a long while.

Not only does the person with multiple sclerosis go through a process of adjustment, but the intimate others in his or her life must do so, too. The rate and intensity with which the ill person, family members, and friends adapt, however, may differ, and communication and other aspects of their relationships may become strained.

Such was the case for Margaret. "I had been diagnosed with M.S. for six years and my family and I had successfully adjusted to my disability. I was pretty much unaffected except for a need to walk with a cane and occasional hand tremors. We proceeded with our lives as if the M.S. was simply an unfortunate accident that left me with a serious leg injury but nothing more.

"Then one morning, while washing up in the bathroom, I felt dizzy and, looking in the mirror, my vision was blurry. I went back to bed and when I tried to get up it seemed as if my body just didn't work anymore. The next day, Eric, my husband, took me to the hospital where I underwent ACTH treatment.* Although my dizziness went away and my vision recovered, when I left

---

*ACTH, adreno-corticotrophic hormone, is a synthetic form of a chemical normally made by the pituitary gland, which stimulates the adrenal gland to produce more steroidal products. It is usually administered over a ten- to fourteen-day period, either by an intravenous drip or by intramuscular injections. The goal of the treatment is to reduce inflammation and immunologic abnormalities. It is most often used when an exacerbation either does not remit in reasonable time or progressively worsens.

the hospital I was in a wheelchair, which I have not given up since.

"It was obviously a very discouraging shock for all of us," Margaret continues. "We felt as if we were starting all over again. The children were very frightened. We all were. We were fortunate that we knew many of the facts of M.S., but the sudden worsening of my condition was in some ways harder to bear than the original diagnosis. After all, at that time we were able to say that the effect of the illness upon me was minimal. I would be able to continue all my roles with simply a degree of inconvenience.

"Although we knew of the potential for greater disability, we said it was not likely to happen to us. We had been fired upon by a bullet of fate and barely grazed. It was doubtful a second bullet would hit us so squarely so soon. Clearly, those were wishful hopes rather than realistic assessments.

"This time I plunged into a depression far deeper than any I had before. I felt as if I couldn't be sure of anything—not my body, not my reactions, not my thoughts. And if I couldn't be sure of me, how could I be sure of anyone else. I had always assumed Eric would be there for me; now I wondered what he really thought or felt. What if he didn't want to live with a cripple? And maybe the kids really hated me because I couldn't do the usual stuff with them. They said they loved me, but could I be sure?

"Pretty soon I started to act toward them as if what I feared was true. I believed that if they were to leave me, I had better learn how to be alone. I withdrew. I took all my natural instincts to reach out and be warm and shut them away. I didn't want to be hurt or to need anybody. I felt angry and cheated by fate. I must have been quite a picture: a scared, bitter woman stuck in a wheelchair. I feel quite badly now, thinking what I must have put everyone through.

"Now I think that if the first attack had disabled me I would have coped with it much better. I guess it's like climbing a mountain. If you start out and there's a snowstorm, right away you just stop and that's it. But to be near the summit and then to be halted by a storm after you've put out so much effort and tasted victory, that must be so much worse. And to have it happen again and again—God, that's terrible. I kept thinking there must be a terrible God for such a thing to happen."

Eric continues their story. "I think we both felt defeated. The exacerbation was a horrible blow. After the original diagnosis, we had put our parents and friends and our own minds at ease and we had stuffed whatever doubts or fears we had way in the back. Now the possibility that we could never know if or when even worse could happen robbed us of any security we felt.

"As Margaret said, she became quite depressed and pulled away from all of us. I was angry at her for being so sick, I suppose, but also for letting me down emotionally. I expected that she could hold it together just as she had done several years before. The more she pulled away from the kids and me, the more I wanted to let her stew in her own juices.

"Our social life halted. Margaret was too depressed to see anybody and I wasn't going to put out any effort. Eventually our friends stopped reaching out as we gave them nothing back. We were drenched in self-pity. She would sit staring at the walls and dozing a lot, and I would be in the TV room or hanging out with the kids—more to avoid Margaret than to offer them anything constructive. Our whole home was freezing emotionally.

"Fortunately, before either one of us said or did things we'd really regret, our minister called to say how much he'd missed us at church. He had been in touch before to express sympathy and concern for Margaret. This time, however, he came over and sat down with us. He was quite insightful and got a good sense of both the despair we were feeling and the crisis in our marriage."

Margaret continues, "He was very straight with us. He said God did not give us more suffering than we could bear. We had two choices: to give in and die emotionally, or to survive. And we were very close to going under. He said I was close to suicide and Eric was close to leaving. Those would have been unforgivable sins to commit against our families and ourselves. It was possible, he said, to draw back from the brink, but we would have to work hard, very hard. With God's grace and with help from a counselor, he thought we could heal the suffering we had inflicted on ourselves and each other. Perhaps, he said, the illness was an opportunity to rekindle the love and purpose we had once found in our lives and marriage."

Margaret and Eric did go to a psychotherapist, but they were unable to close the chasm that had opened between them. While the process of separation and divorce was long and painful, they did, for the sake of the children, manage to maintain the respect for each other that had once been at the center of their marriage. It was more difficult for either of them to recover the straight-forward confidence in life they once held. Their natural optimism became heavily shaded with a sense of the tragic. And over time this was transformed into a sense of compassion for those less fortunate than they.

"It became clear to me," says Margaret, "that much of what I had seen in my depression was true. There was very little that was sure in life. We had taken so much for granted. Because I didn't know when anything might happen—an exacerbation, more illness, an accident—I felt a great need to be of use. I was hung up with wanting to have a purpose, to justify the gift of my life. I praised God for the opportunity given me to get out of myself. With my body confined in a wheelchair, I felt my soul take wing.

"I took courses both at school and at home. I enrolled in some home-based, independent-study college programs and got training and a degree in counseling. I have my own practice and work with several agencies. I've had several exacerbations since that first one. I have become more physically disabled, and my sight has become severely curtailed. Yet with each blow, I feel as if I have become even more in touch with the most important values and more able to listen to each individual's suffering. I am," says Margaret, "more whole even as my body is less free."

Margaret's movement from denial to anger and depression to acceptance and transcendence was neither a short nor easy path. With every exacerbation she was emotionally knocked down, but then she'd pick herself up again with ever more force and conviction. Her pattern is typical of many people with multiple sclerosis. Although observers can hardly believe that people may feel better about themselves and their lives as their illness worsens, it is often the case.

People, however, differ in the ease and time it takes for them to travel the journey from initial shock to acclimation, from denial to acceptance to getting on with the rest of one's life.

The denial stage can be punctuated with shock and disbelief. Surrounded by images of youthfulness and the triumphant technology of modern medicine, we believe we are immune to illness. Our friends and ourselves—twenty, thirty, forty years old—members of the fitness generation, are filled with the energy and drive of people with places to go, things to do, careers to build, families to raise, and dreams to make happen. How could we be stopped cold, suddenly, in our tracks by something we can't see, maybe never heard of, and, certainly, never expected? It's hard to believe that *it* is happening to *you*.

Roger, a young architect, remembers cheerfully greeting visitors to his hospital room with the full facts about his initial diagnosis. "My bed was loaded with books, medical journals, and blocks of paper. I was designing what I called 'ideal access conditions for the handicapped population.' I would tell people that my diagnosis made me realize how much people in wheelchairs needed my help in the movement for improved access. I did not identify myself, personally, with the disabled, but I appreciated their plight more by being exposed to their difficulties on the ward."

Roger's M.S. went into remission directly after his hospitalization. His legs were no longer numb and his weakness virtually disappeared. He was able to return to work and he did so, armed with a false optimism. Roger remained in this initial stage of denial for a long time; it was nearly two years before he experienced any additional symptoms.

Roger's wife, Theresa, however, did not deny what was going on. Like Roger, she educated herself about the disease and soon began to feel angry about the diagnosis and frustrated with Roger's naïveté. "I would tell Roger, 'Please, let's make some contingency plans in case you aren't able to continue to work. What if you can't commute in a couple of years? What if anything happens to your memory or your concentration? Let's think about any changes we can make now that might help your work situation later.' "

Roger refused to focus on any of these issues. "I'd tell Theresa that she was a worrier, that she didn't have a positive attitude. I refused to discuss any of what I considered her negative plans. They had nothing to do with my future. I was convinced that my case was, and would remain, mild."

Roger believed that he was more frustrated with Theresa than with his M.S. He felt vulnerable when she expressed her concerns. He used his wife as the scapegoat for his problems, blaming her for trying to break down his defenses. He felt vulnerable when she expressed her concern.

By the time Roger had his next attack, Theresa was already accepting what a diagnosis of multiple sclerosis meant for their lives. She was understandably anxious about the unpredictability of the disease, but she remained realistic about their future together and loyal to Roger. Roger, in contrast, was exceedingly angry and fearful about his new symptoms. He could no longer deny the correctness of the original diagnosis. His doctors did not seem overly concerned about him. They treated him as if another attack were expected.

Roger was furious. "I'd demand answers from my physicians and my wife. 'Why is this happening to me?' I wasn't meant to be sick, I thought. I had too many plans for the future." Roger's anger was a good sign that he was entering the second stage of adjustment. Fortunately, at the same time, Theresa had gone a long way in accepting the new realities with which they were faced. She was convinced that they could continue their life together in a manner no less satisfying, though in some ways different, than before.

Theresa's commitment, and the competent medical and psychological support Roger and she received, assisted this couple in achieving a normal adjustment. Roger was soon able to proceed to the next, more accepting phase. Yet due to anxiety about future attacks and the hope that naturally accompanied each remission, Roger continued to maintain: "This last exacerbation may be my last. Who knows?"

As Roger began to accept his M.S. and the impact it had upon his life, he began to appreciate people and activities that for years he had taken for granted. "The second time I was admitted to the hospital, I wrote out a gratitude list and gave it to Theresa. At the top was my thankfulness for her ability and courage to confront me about my denial of my illness and my gratitude that I was able to love her again. I couldn't have blamed her if she had left me after all the crap I gave her about her 'negative thinking.' "

Roger also began to feel more comfortable with the feelings of dependency that accompanied his M.S. diagnosis. A shift in roles and tasks at home often meant that Theresa had to take care of the physical chores that used to be Roger's primary responsibilities. In response, Roger became more of an administrative personality. For example, when they were remodeling a bathroom, Theresa learned how to tile, while Roger negotiated with the contractors and scheduled the work time necessary to complete the job. Their identities complemented each other in a new and healthy way. The concept of man's work versus woman's work was no longer a viable one in this truly cooperative household.

Roger's friendships in the community also changed as a result of his M.S., and a major portion of the adjustment process involved separating sincere from superficial friends. The latter group often loses interest in anyone who cannot keep up with activities. Roger had invested many years in sports teams and neighborhood projects with the same group of young men, and he had a difficult time adjusting to their lack of phone calls and general interest in him.

"I had to continue to value myself," Roger remembers, "to recognize that their separation and distance was due to their shallowness and reflective of their problems with communication. Yet I did feel different from my more active former friends. I was no longer free to join in the sports and games I still loved. And to my chagrin, these losses that were so important to me did not seem to matter at all to so many others."

Anyone who has the complications of a chronic disease or disability has difficulty making plans. Activities that were formerly anticipated with relish are now regarded as less achievable. Roger's case is, unfortunately, not unusual. Very often, acquaintances and even loved ones do not understand enough to help someone with multiple sclerosis along. Some friends do become more available when an individual has adjusted to his or her illness enough to feel comfortable with a group despite an inability to participate in the same way as before.

"People I played tennis with didn't call me to ask for a game, and I felt too useless and resentful to get together with them. Finally, I took the risk of inviting myself over when a couple of guys I knew were playing tennis. I'd sit in the shade, kibitz about their game, and we'd all cool off afterward. We all realized that our neglect of each other was motivated by embarrassment and confusion. We found we could still be together, although we couldn't 'do' together in the same way as before."

Old ways of assessing oneself are replaced by new,

more realistic ways in the adapting/adjusting stage. Perspective broadens as the person with M.S. reemerges into society. He or she is better able to see the talents and strengths that are not connected with illness. M.S. becomes part of one's life, but not the whole of it. Though symptoms may always be present, an individual makes coping with his illness secondary to meeting his goals in life.

It is worth repeating that adjustment to multiple sclerosis and its unpredictable course is not a once-and-for-all event never to be faced again. Active problem solving replaces the defense of denial that was present in the early stages of adjustment. Yet when symptoms increase and new demands must be met, shock, anger, and depression are aroused once more. The whole business is ongoing.

Nevertheless, the first phase of the continuum from denial to adjustment is typically the most difficult one. The irrevocable fact of the diagnosis is admitted. The support of family and friends tested and enlisted, the possibility of change in career and life-style discussed, the fear of disease and death confronted. Something is created in oneself after those first dark nights that provides a source of determination and solace, of courage and gratitude for the journey, however rocky, that lies ahead.

Probably the most important ingredients in the adjustment process are the personal coping resources a person brings to his encounter with multiple sclerosis and the support of family, friends, and community. No two people adjust the same way. No two people experience the effects of this illness in the same manner. Yet adjustment can be successful and a satisfying life is available.

Roger states this most poignantly when he says, "Theresa and I do not know what the future may bring. But then, no one does. We may have to deal with big changes in the future and, strangely, that could be an advantage. After all, Theresa and I no longer see ourselves as invulnerable. We know that the Sword of Damocles could fall on any one of us at any time.

"So we draw up plans for the future and, at the same time, take advantage of each day as much as possible. Without this illness, we might have taken too much for granted. And that would be a shame in a world as wondrous as this one."

❖ 7 ❖

Is My Thinking Okay?

MULTIPLE SCLEROSIS STRIKES young adults in their physical and intellectual prime. It hits during the most productive period of one's life—at the end of schooling and in the early work years. These are the years when one's ability to think and solve problems is most essential. Yet while M.S. can mildly impair complex thought processes, the potential for alteration in one's ability to think and remember may be an aspect of the disease. An individual with M.S. is typically more aware of the overt physical symptoms commonly associated with M.S. Subtle cognitive changes may also begin to occur in less than half of those with the disease. These are rarely severe problems.

People with M.S. can begin to have difficulties performing tasks that had previously been automatic. For reasons that no physical examination can answer, someone with this illness can make errors recalling job responsibilities they may have known for many years. It is perplexing as well that there is no correlation between changes in cognitive functioning and the severity of other physical impairments.

Fortunately, one can usually successfully adapt to these cognitive deficits through learning style and readjustment. It is helpful to note, however, that people who compensate for their weaknesses of coordination and mobility may fear that they are unable to master mental tasks. You may wonder if the subtle changes are related to demyelination or reactive depression. In truth, it could be either.

Janet's husband, Robert, began to lose patience with her "fender bender" accidents, which were occurring all too often. "She would have the same story each time," Robert relates. "She would be stopped at a red light in a line of traffic, talking to the children. When the light turned green, she'd accelerate and then have to stop quickly to avoid hitting the car in front of her. But hit them she did—at least three times in as many months. The fourth time, she bumped a pedestrian crossing the street. Fortunately, no one was injured."

Janet continues the story. "Robert was really angry with me. He said I was irresponsible and that I was costing us a lot of money and him a lot of worry. We agreed that I'd put in extra hours at work to make up for the cash we were losing from my accidents. I started thinking of myself as a scatterbrain and I thought I could at least take financial responsibility for my actions."

Neither Janet nor Robert connected her difficulties estimating speed and distance and her slower response time with her M.S. Janet's symptoms had not changed and she remained only minimally disabled. Although she complained occasionally of feeling tired or drained after shopping, she continued to carry on all her home responsibilities quite effectively.

"The additional work load proved to be too much,"

Janet says. "I started to make errors at work I had never made before, and I became quite fatigued at home. I stumbled more often and even dropped a dish or two. Although our neurologist told us that there was no obvious change in my strength or balance, Robert and I were concerned enough to consult a counselor who had experience working with people with M.S. When she heard our story, including the account of all my accidents, she referred me right away to a neuropsychologist."

After hearing of Janet's recent mishaps, the neuropsychologist proposed giving Janet some tests to evaluate her level of problem solving and memory abilities. In addition, in the case of people with M.S. as well as with many other chronic diseases and aging itself, it is always wise to pose the question: Is the change in thinking and memory a result of damage to the nervous system, or is it a consequence of the significant emotional stresses associated with the illness? The tests that a neuropsychologist provides can reveal cognitive deficits that are missed by even the most complete physical examination.

The testing showed that Janet's thinking was quite good. But like many people with multiple sclerosis, she did poorly on measures that were in part dependent on touch and visual recall. These were exactly the skills demanded for automobile driving. Janet's frequent accidents were a result of her inability to adequately judge distances between cars and coordinate her acceleration with her perception of those distances.

The results happily demonstrated that Janet's capacity for attention and concentration was not impaired. She was as bright as ever and she still had a very good memory. Also, emotional stress was not to blame for her brain damage.

Robert was grateful and somewhat embarrassed by

these findings. "I thought that because Janet's symptoms had not changed for years that her M.S. was 'under control' and certainly could not be responsible for her current difficulties." He was learning to appreciate the subtle but important changes in brain and behavior that accompany neurological disease.

Janet was pleased that she knew the source of her weaknesses. She had always been a logical, practical thinker, and she felt comfortable with the compensation techniques the neuropsychologist taught her. "I learned to talk to myself, just quiet enough so no one would hear, about distance and acceleration. I'd say: 'There's seven feet between our cars . . . now let's start slowly . . . be careful . . . now a little more pressure on the gas. . . .' I used a cookbook approach to driving, which was just like the way I first learned at driving school. I took it slow and easy and I did just fine.

"It was also invaluable for Robert and me to discover together that, as always, there were some difficulties to M.S. that we had not appreciated and that we could continue to meet the challenge."

Though people with multiple sclerosis show the greatest decline in areas that involve movement, coordination, and visual skills, they can also experience a degree of impairment in perceiving what they are hearing. Sometimes it may become difficult to perceive individual speech sounds as well as to remember and respond to rhythms.

Often, persons complain of dizziness or vertigo. Such was Gwen's experience. In the middle of the school day, just as she was preparing her kindergarten youngsters for lunch, she began to feel dizzy, and had to immediately sit down to rest. It appeared to her as if the entire room was spinning around. She felt she no longer could trust herself to accompany the children to the lunchroom or supervise them during recess. She was concerned that her thinking was impaired.

Mr. Gilmore, Gwen's principal, was quite helpful. It seemed that his wife had many such attacks, and they found the answer to her problems at the Eye and Ear Infirmary in their capital city. "I would gladly make an appointment for you to see her doctor," he offered. "The sooner your symptoms are cleared up, the better we will all feel. They are uncomfortable, but they do not impact upon your ability to make decisions or how you relate to the children. Your thinking is certainly intact."

Gwen's appointment was made for the following week, and in the meantime her symptoms repeatedly returned. As a result, she required rides to school and regular coverage for her class. Dr. Singer was kind and forceful. "The obvious diagnosis for this type of attack," he explained, "is middle-ear infection or Ménière's disease. I have just the medication to control it." Gwen was relieved to hear him add, "It has nothing to do with your teaching ability."

The prescribed medication and extra rest appeared to lessen Gwen's symptoms. In addition, the fatigue that she had become acutely aware of also disappeared. She was generally symptom-free for about two years. After that time, however, she again had to visit the audiologist. Though she no longer felt dizzy and lightheaded, her ears were bothered in a different way. She had a hyper-acuity of hearing; the slightest sound seemed to jar her in a painful manner.

Dr. Singer, puzzled by this new symptom, decided to refer Gwen to a local neurologist. "This is not typically seen in Ménière's disease," he explained. "It sounds like something else to me." Gwen was then given her diagnosis of multiple sclerosis.

In addition, memory can be affected when a person's

attention is not specifically focused. This more frequently occurs when alertness is compromised by competing thoughts. At such times, an individual may be described by companions as having "a one-track mind," able to concentrate in only one direction at a time.

Memory can also be affected by fatigue. It is often difficult for anyone, particularly those with M.S., to remain visually alert at night. The darkness, as well as approaching car lights, can be confusing and frustrating to someone already exhausted by chronic illness. One can even lose one's way home.

Kenneth, who had been diagnosed with M.S. for the past three years, had taken the same route home for the five years he and his wife, Lucy, had lived near the expressway. He used to joke that the car ran on automatic pilot on the commute home. "One evening, however," Ken relates, "I found myself wandering around on the roads of a neighboring town. I excused my behavior as simply a result of taking the wrong exit. I asked for directions and eventually arrived home, where Lucy and I laughed about my absentmindedness.

"The next time that we drove and I got lost it was not so comical. We were on our way to a party at the home of some old friends and we arrived over an hour late. We were embarrassed explaining to our hosts, people whose home we had visited so many times before, that we had left in plenty of time, but had merely become lost en route.

"I finally agreed to a neuropsychological evaluation," Ken admits, "when I found myself walking around an office building one day, unable to recall in which office a major appointment was scheduled. My secretary had apparently mentioned the number to me while I was looking at blueprints I was to deliver. In the past, I would always jot down the address in my notebook in case

I forgot, but I didn't even think to do that. This was an extremely important appointment and I was very bothered by my sloppiness. I figured it had to be something medical."

Ken and Lucy were concerned about the pending evaluation. They imagined all kinds of negative findings. What if he could no longer work or follow Lucy's train of thought or conversations? "I was so anxious that I stumbled over my words. I had difficulty recalling the names of people with whom I had worked for years. And I was getting very upset over the slightest change in plans—certainly more than what was deserved."

Ken relaxed considerably, however, after merely a few minutes into the testing. He found himself relating well to the examiner, and feeling challenged by the interesting material. Even before hearing the results, he perceived that he had done well on most of the tests administered to him. The neuropsychologist explained to him that his current intellectual abilities were in the same range as before he had been diagnosed with multiple sclerosis. He could still learn and process new facts and information, function effectively at work and at home, and relate to other people as well as he had formerly.

However, he did need to focus directly on situations in order to master and remember them. He could no longer rely upon being able to pick up information incidentally, nor was he able to absorb material as casually as before. Ken had to remember to pay attention to what he wanted to know. If he was too tired or given many directions at one time, he could easily lose a portion. He would become flooded and confused about details.

In addition, when Ken became tense or flustered and overly anxious about his memory, his thinking skills slipped. Testing showed that his disturbances in memory were based more upon his fearfulness about what M.S. could do than the actual physical impact of the illness.

"We were both quite relieved by the results of the evaluation," Lucy remembers. "It wasn't too difficult for us to come up with some coping strategies now that we knew what we were dealing with. It was very reassuring to find that there was so much more Ken could continue to do, and that we could compensate for his areas of weakness. The peace of mind we both received from the evaluation was well worth the four-hour investment of time and energy."

Multiple sclerosis, in contrast to many other neurological diseases, is responsible for only mild impairments, if any at all, in grasping the nature of a problem. The ability to get to the root of what other people say and mean also remains intact. Consequently, Louise, our psychiatrist friend from Chapter 1, appeared to have a relatively benign time adjusting her M.S. to her career. She was able, as before her illness, to recall what her patients told her and offer helpful interpretations. Indeed, at times her own adjustment to chronic illness contributed to her ability to serve her patients.

Louise also gained insight into her strengths and weaknesses. "I've spent the last few years coming to terms with my newfound deficits. When one of my friends asked me to help her decorate her house and visualize what alternative arrangements of furnishings and space would look like, I had to laugh and tell her to look elsewhere for design advice.

"I was always aware that my talents were not artistic, and since my M.S., that is even more the case. But it still does not stop me from trying out new things. I just don't get overly concerned with results.

"My clients, of course, appreciate my ability to listen,

analyze, and talk. They're often surprised by how much I remember of what they tell me. I think everyone is better or worse in certain areas, and the M.S. simply made me more aware than most people of where my talents lay. I don't waste time wishing I could do what I can't. I try to use what I do have as fully as I am able."

The basis for adaptation and adjustment to changes in thinking and memory is a thorough assessment by a qualified professional. Armed with this information, a person with M.S. and the important people in his life are equipped to cope successfully with problems in brain behavior.

The key is in teaching people to better understand how to capitalize on their strengths and compensate for their weaknesses. Some persons who have difficulty with planning and organization may have to make lists and designate very consistent and structured ways to accomplish these tasks. Persons who have difficulty concentrating may require short intervals to accomplish things, or a relative or spouse to periodically monitor and refocus them. M.S. persons who have problems with directionality, reading graphs, charts, pictures, etc., could learn to talk their way through tasks in a detailed, repetitive manner.

In general, M.S. persons have the most difficulty and show some dysfunction in all tasks that require motor performance. Their motor speed and coordination is decreased. In contrast, little or no compromise is seen in patients' abilities to respond to verbal information, comprehension of verbal communication, or problem solving. Multiple sclerosis does not usually interfere with people's abilities to use verbal reasoning in problem solving.

❖ 8 ❖

Can We Still Make Love?

MULTIPLE SCLEROSIS CAN MAKE sexual expression and lovemaking more problematic in a variety of ways. M.S. often has neurological effects upon sexual function that may be present even when other functions are minimally impaired. As a result, when a diagnosis of multiple sclerosis is made, there may already be a history of frustration, conflict, uncertainty, and depression about this vital area. Thus, a diagnosis may provide both a sense of relief that there could be a physical cause to these disturbing changes as well as some apprehension that these difficulties may not be easily solved. A major challenge then is to open lines of communication that may have become blocked.

"In the two or three years preceding my diagnosis," confides Frank, "I had increasing difficulty maintaining an erection and more frequent episodes of failing to have one at all. This was extremely frustrating to Bonnie and me. After each unsuccessful attempt at lovemaking we'd try to analyze what went wrong, what we could do differently, what was going on psychologically, and so on. And soon enough, we'd start blaming each other and end up not only physically unsatisfied, but emotionally distant.

"When I was finally diagnosed," Frank continues, "I actually welcomed it with some relief. At least I had a reason for my dysfunction. It wasn't all in my head and it wasn't due to some unconscious anger Bonnie or I had toward each other. It took a lot of the personal and emotional charge off the issue, and we thought we would be able to approach what to do about it more rationally."

Frank and Bonnie were fortunate that they were able to keep communicating with each other despite the enormous pressure and anxiety they both felt. Although sex was an important aspect of their relationship, they did not allow a lack of satisfaction in that area to create a permanent gulf of anger and despair. They were committed to ways of sharing that included, but were not limited to, sexual expression.

For some couples, a diagnosis of M.S. serves only to inhibit them from talking with each other about sexual issues they now believe hopeless to resolve. They may feel as if the relationship itself, rather than simply the sexual aspect of it, is at risk. To couples who are coping with the shock of diagnosis and the strain of new and frightening demands, to be concerned with sexuality seems an indulgence they can ill-afford. In fact, sexual issues often serve as lightning rods that attract and deflect emotions from more fundamental conflicts and questions in the relationship.

"Once we recognized that my M.S. was the cause of my sexual difficulties," Frank continues, "Bonnie and I were able to talk more easily. But I still felt guilty that she was not able to have the kind of sexual relationship I felt she, and we, deserved. I even suggested, half-jokingly, that she have affairs so she wouldn't be deprived of a full sex life because of my illness. Having a diagnosis solved some of the problems of our sexual relationship, but it also created some new ones."

Bonnie also felt guilty about her attitude toward Frank and their sexual difficulties. "There was no question I felt resentment toward Frank because his M.S. kept us from having the kind of sexual relationship I wanted and we were working toward prior to his illness. And I felt even worse when I fantasized about affairs because, and in spite, of his jokes. I knew he would be crushed if I did have one, and I also knew I couldn't handle the emotional and physical splits that an affair would create. I loved Frank. I wanted sex with him, not a surrogate. And what was doubly frustrating was that the relief from tension that sex usually provides under conditions of stress was unavailable. We both felt crummy."

The tough experience Frank and Bonnie were having with sex began to seep into other areas of their relationship and their personal lives. They began to pull back from touching and holding because they did not want to be pulled into a pattern of sexual response and failure that promised only anxiety and frustration. The reassurance and bonding that physical closeness provided began to disappear from their lives. They avoided each other in the evenings and began to fantasize about relationships with other people in which intimacy, not sex, was primary. The emotional connection they could, and once did, offer each other began to fray.

Frank and Bonnie had to come to terms with the disappointment and sorrow each felt as individuals and as a couple for the dire change in the sexual aspect of their relationship before they could begin to rebuild the sexual and sensual elements of their partnership. Although their pattern of sexual conduct would change, their lives could still be rich with sexual satisfaction. The first step, however, was communication.

"We loved each other so much that our moving apart when Frank was ill just hurt us terribly," remembers Bonnie. "And we felt helpless. Before, when we had arguments, we could use our bodies to heal the splits between us. Now sex wasn't available in the same easy way. We were very sad."

"We decided we needed to speak with a therapist about our relationship and coping with my M.S.," Frank adds. "I felt a lot of embarrassment talking about my sexual difficulties with my doctors and we also felt that our sexuality was best helped in the context of our whole relationship.

"Our therapist was very helpful. She suggested we speak to a neurologist to get information about sexual response and M.S. and the physiology of arousal. She said having that knowledge would be helpful in understanding and accepting the changes that result from M.S. and appreciating the many opportunities for sexual fulfillment still open to us."

"I wouldn't describe the sessions as easy," states Bonnie, "because we felt we had been sexually competent prior to Frank's illness. Now we were sexual beginners. And while we anticipated the possibility of a reawakened sex life, we also were apprehensive about exploring and experimenting in an area that had been so fraught with tension. But Frank and I were committed to improving our relationship."

The impact of multiple sclerosis upon an individual's sexual response and a couple's sexual interactions may create the need for readjustments, both psychological and sexual, that range from minor to significant. The taken-for-granted moves and movements that once brought pleasure and excitement may no longer do so. Partners who once knew from trial and error what each enjoyed or found uncomfortable, may avoid sexual activity rather than communicate openly about physical intimacies and performance concerns. For most people, even those with satisfying sexual relationships, feelings of guilt, shame, and embarrassment may be associated with sexual and sensual activity and enjoyment.

"One thing that was pointed out to me," says Frank, "was my denial of how bad I felt about my sexual difficulties. Although I wouldn't admit it, I felt as if I were less of a man and a lover. I also didn't understand how Bonnie's pulling back was her attempt to not pressure me into performing, to give me time to work out my feelings about my problem. I took her withdrawal as disapproval and a lack of interest in me. And since she did not appear eager, I wasn't going to push myself on her."

Bonnie continues the story. "I was also denying the anger and frustration I felt with Frank. I thought I was in a bind. At the same time I wanted him to do something about his problems, I felt as if I were making his attempts to cope with M.S. more difficult by burdening him with something as trivial as our sex life. He was under enough pressure, so I backed away. At the same time, his lack of sexual interest led me to think that I was not fulfilling my role as companion and comforter as well as I might. I felt guilty about being concerned with sex when something as grave and serious as M.S. was happening to us. All in all, we were each feeling worse and worse about ourselves."

At the same time that she was helping Frank and Bonnie take a look at the crosscurrents of anger and guilt, longing and elusion, their therapist helped them to expand their notions of sexuality and the scope of their sexual options. Because sexual intercourse may be less satisfying or more difficult with M.S., couples who avoid it may believe they are missing out on sex itself. In fact, there are many ways of enjoying sexual relationships in which intercourse plays little or no role at all. For those couples whose sexual activity has focused on intercourse as the goal, M.S. may encourage them to experiment with a wider variety of giving and receiving physical pleasure.

As with food, reading, sports, and just about any area of personal enjoyment, the ways and means of sexual satisfaction ought to be a matter of individual preference. The freedom from narrow definitions of sexual propriety or confining sex roles has benefited no group so much as the ill or disabled. We know that both men and women enjoy being "aggressive" or "passive" in sexual encounters and that orgasms are as often or more commonly a result of manual or oral stimulation as by intercourse for many people. When couples begin to share with one another the similarities and differences of what feels good and comfortable to them, they are often delightfully surprised by each other's fantasies and revelations.

"We found," relates Bonnie, "that we had to relearn for ourselves and reeducate each other about what we wanted and felt good about sexually. For Frank, the holding and cuddling that had previously led straight to intercourse now became something he desired for its own sake. I also became more accepting of his need for oral sex when his capacity for genital performance was more limited.

"It's kind of funny, actually. Our sexual styles began to shade more toward each other's. Frank began to appreciate more the warm reassurance of touch, and I was more open to finding sexual alternatives for our enjoyment. Sometimes we'd get frustrated or irritated if something that seemed to be okay one week didn't feel as pleasant the next. But when we treated our experimentation as an opportunity to get reacquainted, even to put some exciting romance into our relationship, we'd relax again."

There are ways in which intercourse may be possible despite changes in erectile function. Some men find certain positions more stimulating. There are techniques in which some vaginal entry is achieved that may be enjoyable. And penile implants are increasingly used as an alternative to permanent organic erectile dysfunction. For men and women with thigh spasms, which make intercourse painful or uncomfortable, certain medications or altering positions may be useful.

We recommend that people who want to investigate these various alternatives speak with their physician, a patient service worker from their local chapter of the National M.S. Society, or their personal counselor. At times, counselors from local agencies that work with spinal cord patients or disabled veterans may be helpful in this regard.

We strongly recommend that everyone with a sexual concern related to M.S. read *Sexuality & Multiple Sclerosis*, by Michael Barrett. It may be obtained from the National Multiple Sclerosis Society, 733 Third Avenue, New York, NY 10017-3288. The booklet contains an excellent bibliography and is a source of some of the information in this chapter.

As with any activity and M.S., the fatigue factor can play an inhibiting role in regard to sex. It can affect interest in initiating sexual encounters as well as responsiveness to stimulation. Feeling obliged to have sex when one is physically exhausted is a surefire way to weaken its appeal in the long run.

Roy and Tricia had been married for twelve years when Tricia was diagnosed with multiple sclerosis. The only constant symptom she was aware of in those first few years was an imposing fatigue. By the time Roy returned home from work in the evening, she was stretched out on the sofa trying to rest. The process of bathing her two sons (ages two and four) grew more exhausting to her each week.

"We would begin dinner each evening after Tricia had had a short rest," Roy explains. "She would then have enough energy to sit at the table with us for a full hour. We would be able to catch up with each other. It was great to talk, laugh, and have fun with the boys until our stomachs were full."

"The evening would continue so well up to that point," Tricia continues. "Roy would put Jeff and Sam to bed as I completed the dishes. Just as he came downstairs, fully relaxed and ready for our private time together, I would become exhausted and want to collapse in bed, alone."

"I often became so disappointed, I'd be turned off almost as quickly as I'd be turned on," Roy adds. "People advise communicating about everything but that. I became so disappointed at Tricia's fatigue, and yet felt honestly guilty for feeling this way when she had so much more to be concerned about, that I could not bear to broach this delicate subject with her."

It is essential for some couples to compromise the spontaneity of sexual encounters and be sensitive to the fatigue factor. Improved timing can often make all the difference between dreading or enjoying the relaxed togetherness that physical closeness can bring. Opening communication for an honest sharing of feelings can help both members of the couple understand how much they both need intimacy and how much they both miss the reassurance of being needed—and together.

Roy and Tricia finally rearranged their schedules so that they had an opportunity to come together in bed early in the mornings. The evenings became the time for physical affection—hugging, holding, and feeling close.

Sex, like all forms of physical activity we enjoy, is both energizing and relaxing. If you are going to feel worse as a result of engaging in sex when you are at low ebb physically, let it go.

Up until the time he was diagnosed with M.S., Nicholas and Isabel had had a good marriage and an enjoyable sex life. "My disability was moderate," Nicholas points out, "primarily affecting my ability to walk without fatigue and to play the sports I loved. I continued to work as before, but by the time I came home in the evening I was tired and irritable. I would get angry at Isabel for small things and I would then feel quite badly about it. I began going to bed earlier than I ever had before.

"It was obvious, although unspoken by either of us, that I was less interested in sex than before. I simply avoided it by going to bed. I know that Isabel was quite frustrated, but I told her that if I stayed up any later when I was already so tired it would affect my work the next day. I know now that although the fatigue was real and, perhaps, a symptom of my M.S., it was also the result of the depression I was feeling and the difficulty I was having coming to terms with my illness.

"Finally," Nicholas continues, "the situation became intolerable for both of us. There was no physical reason we couldn't make love, and we each really longed to enjoy each other as before, but Isabel didn't want to pressure me. At her suggestion we contacted the M.S. Society, which referred us to a family counselor who works with people with chronic illness. She helped us talk about our feelings, which were mutual: We both wanted to reestablish sexual relations in a caring and relaxed manner.

"We set up a schedule that involved changing our rest times and sex times from what they were before. The compromises we made in bedtime, waking time, and nap time were insignificant compared to getting back to the mutual pleasure we gave each other."

Sometimes, however, letting go becomes a habit. People avoid sex simply because it seems easier to do so than to plan zestful and restful lovemaking. It is wise to consider whether you want to make sex a lesser priority than other activities that you include in your life. Sex need not be a spur-of-the-moment thing. Its spontaneity emerges in the affectionate interplay of two people intimately sharing themselves. Scheduling sex for when your energy is highest, making arrangements for the children to be away, taking a nap before your encounter can all contribute to a morning or afternoon delight.

It is much easier to deal with the blows to self-esteem and self-confidence that may arise from sexual difficulties within the context of a relationship than to face the potential rejection and isolation that single persons with M.S. fear and, on occasion, meet. Many single people must overcome the hindrances to social involvement before addressing sexual concerns. Anxieties about incontinence, fatigue, physical and sensory disturbances all may serve to prevent a person with a chronic illness or disability from initiating the interactions that may lead to more intimate situations.

As Rachel recounts, "I was afraid that if I did ever get into a more serious dating arrangement, all my symptoms would become exaggerated and highly visible. In public settings I already imagined that everybody was looking at and pitying me. Even people I didn't know were my audience.

"Once I was alone with someone, I thought my partner would notice a lot about my body and my gestures that pointed to the fact that I was ill. My clothes and my playing it cool were a kind of protection from acknowledging both my physical limitations and my sexuality.

"Refraining from sex and tighter commitments also kept me from getting too involved with people. I feared some would leave me once they became more aware of the curtailments that M.S. put into my life. Others I thought I would leave because of my guilt at 'seducing' them into a relationship in which they were bound to be unhappy. I felt very unattractive and thought I appealed only to men who needed a wounded bird. Normal men would not want a physical relationship with me. I thought good sex was only for the trim and slim workout types.

"My counselor suggested," Rachel goes on, "that some of my difficulty with establishing rapport and following through with men was not simply a result of my M.S. but a pattern of relating that predated my diagnosis. I had to admit that was true, but I also believe M.S. exacerbated the issue.

"She also thought that it was better to initiate and develop friendships out of which sexual opportunities might evolve than to pursue the typical dating game where how someone looks is more important at first than who they are."

As Rachel points out, "Since my physical condition made typical singles spots difficult to attend, I looked for other places where I could meet people. I thought of various political and volunteer activities and continuing education courses. I wanted to get to know people by doing constructive things with them. I didn't want to feel the pressure to play a socially entrancing role that dating situations often require. I wanted to have time for other people and me to get to know each other."

Rachel was fortunate to meet quite a few men and women of different ages through her participation in community-action projects. Feeling good about herself and more confident about her social strengths, she allowed some of her acquaintanceships with men to evolve into casual dating and a few into more intimate relationships.

Because they had created bonds of friendship before seeking romance, Rachel and her partners were able to communicate fairly well with each other over the anxiety and fears brought about by her M.S. The openness of their discussions enabled them to speak about sexual needs and preferences with relatively little embarrassment. These are the kinds of exchanges in which real emotional intimacy precedes the sexual intimacy that might be beneficial to anyone, with or without chronic illness.

It's also true that some people tire of being "just friends" and want the excitement of sexual pursuit and game playing. For those people, self-confidence and a positive body-image are crucial. Otherwise, they might become particularly disheartened in what is even for physically healthy people a sometimes discouraging adventure.

Whatever one's current style, sex is often an enjoyable

and, for some people, profound activity. What we call sex includes an enormous range of habits, morals, tastes, whims, preferences, positions, partners, responses, and emotions. For most people, the opportunity for sexual satisfaction is enhanced by communication between partners about personal and mutual needs and desires.

Sexuality does not halt with disability. It may continue the same or it may change in its expression. It is not necessary to abandon being sexual simply because one must adapt to physical limitations or the annoying and challenging demands of illness. The pattern of sexual conduct in any relationship does not remain fixed. Whereas many people see nothing unusual in changing their diets over time, eating more or less of this food or that, dining out rather than at home, and learning to cook new dishes, the same people often assume that sex ought to stay the same. It need not.

To be deprived of the opportunity to participate as fully as one wishes in one's sexual life and potential is terrible. But, as is the case with many of those with multiple sclerosis or any chronic illness or disability, obstacles give rise to challenges. These, in their turn, lead to the courageous search for new means of expression. The painter without hands uses toes, the man who cannot speak uses sign language, the woman who cannot run races can still compete in her wheelchair or on crutches. The human spirit in all its forms and forces incessantly seeks new channels from which to pour forth. Who among us does not want to offer and accept love, tenderness, pleasure, and relief? We are all irrevocably sexual.

✦ 9 ✦

Adolescents with M.S.

WHEN MULTIPLE SCLEROSIS STRIKES a person already established in a marriage, family, or career the effect can be devastating. How much more tragic it is when chronic illness afflicts a teenager or young adult. An older individual has the resources of a more fully formed personality and the experience to weather life's disappointments and crises. He can grapple with how he is going to fit M.S. into the existing structure of his life.

A youth, on the other hand, is still trying to master the developmental tasks from which his personality emerges. In addition, rarely has a young person gone through the vicissitudes of life that enable an adult to view even normal and expected difficulties as less than life-ending tragedies. Young people must cope not only with a disease or disability, but with continuing to mature as persons at the same time.

The primary task of an adolescent is to move along toward establishing an identity—a more or less secure sense of who she is, where she stands with her parents and other authority figures, a somewhat realistic idea of what she would like to do with her life, the sort of values she has and the kinds of people she wants to be with, and a feeling of comfort with her body and her sexuality. It is the rare and, probably, imaginary young person that fully attains these goals, but it is possible to take steps toward them, albeit in a two forward, one back manner. A diagnosis of multiple sclerosis can play havoc with this crucial, sometimes turbulent, always exciting process.

"For a long time my parents and I chalked up my stumbles and dropped glasses and plates to teenage awkwardness," recalls Jean. "It was a big joke in the family about how my feet were growing before the rest of my body and that explained my clumsiness. But when I had an attack of double vision, we became very concerned, although we didn't connect the different physical events.

"For a long time both my family and my doctors thought my symptoms were a result of stress or some passing illness, like mononucleosis. Tiredness, vision problems, funny sensations in my arms and legs were all due to one thing or another. I thought I was a real jerk to be complaining about something that was probably only in my head, although my parents told me they believed me. I figured they thought I was just going through a stage or was on drugs or something. I was convinced I must be crazy.

"After all this time had passed, after I'd been to doctors' offices and hospitals, and the doctors said I had multiple sclerosis, I felt really scared. Sure, they and my parents explained it all, but most everything they said just floated right by me. All I remembered were the words 'multiple sclerosis,' a definitely dreaded disease. At least I'm not bonkers, I thought; instead I'll be dead. I saw myself in a wheelchair as some friendless, shriveled-up old lady. I knew no one would want to go out with me, that I'd just be a drag to my friends and a freak at school. I'd be one of those people they tell jokes about, although no one would do it to my face."

Adolescents are typically anxious about their bodies. How their bodies look to others and how they look and feel to themselves is a source of or threat to a positive self-image. The ability to function competently in sports and appear attractive is important to young people of both sexes. Older youth who manage to do one or both are role models for their younger or less-well-endowed peers. Thus, injury or illness may be a profound attack upon one's often shaky search for self-esteem.

Gloria had just turned sixteen when she was diagnosed with M.S. Her parents and close friends had been teasing her for several months about her inability to negotiate through narrow spaces. She was always bumping into pieces of furniture. "At first I was relieved that I really had something to blame my 'clumsiness' on," she admitted to Ronda, her best friend. "My legs would seem to give way at the dumbest times, around home with company, in restaurants, even in school." The relief was, however, short-lived. "It was funny," Gloria continues, "I started to miss the kids' teasing. They didn't say anything, they just stared at me when I bumped into something. I know now that they didn't know what to say, but at the time I was convinced they thought I was weird."

One day after she had tripped, Gloria saw a classmate walk up to the teacher's desk. "I was sure he was talking about me," she explains, "and I started feeling so down."

Soon Gloria started having trouble sleeping, and she complained of losing her appetite. Her parents noticed that their previously well-adjusted daughter seemed to prefer hiding in her bedroom to socializing with friends on weekends. Her mother notes, "She looked sad all the time; even her voice changed. She sounded tense, unexcited."

Gloria had never before shown signs of any mental disorder. There was no history of depression in any of her relatives, yet the psychologist who saw Gloria said that she appeared to be suffering from a reactive depression. He suggested that Gloria meet with him weekly for several sessions in order to help her adjust to her diagnosis. Soon her appetite and sleep habits improved.

Gloria liked this man, who listened to everything she had to say without judging her. As she explained to him, "My parents still think of me as a little kid. They want to know everything I'm thinking so they can correct it." Gloria was describing one of the difficulties all families have in dealing with adolescent children. Parents can no longer be totally involved with their children and be in full authority to "fix any problem." For many parents, even when things are going well, it is difficult to learn that flexibility is necessary in dealing with their teenagers. Parents cannot be "in charge" of their adolescent children as they were able to be over their toddlers. So M.S. makes an already difficult position worse.

"I feel suspended, not like a whole person. I am different from all my friends. I feel like I'm part of a jigsaw puzzle, the piece that doesn't quite fit," Gloria explained to her therapist.

Gloria was most concerned with what the rest of her social set thought of her. She questioned, "How could I relate my plan for the unpredictable? How do I know what course my disease will take?" She admitted to feeling depressed much of the time, and tried to escape from meeting her friends whenever possible. It was an uncomfortable but necessary time to experience. Gloria was in mourning for her past, healthy life. She was experiencing grief. Though this is a painful period, it is an essential one. Grief has an innate healing component. Gloria's parents and close friends had to allow her this intense experience. She required the luxury of her mourning. Though they would have liked to be more involved, it was time for them to stand back.

Luckily, this period did not last long for Gloria; she had a history of good coping strategies. Her self-image had always been fairly intact; though it was obviously shaken by the entire adjustment process, it eventually regained strength. She began to visualize herself in alternate roles, depending on how she was feeling. She, too, was adapting to a more flexible self.

These stages of adjustment to multiple sclerosis obviously differ in people according to what their lives were like prior to M.S. In Gloria's case, her positive past experiences coupled with professional help were beneficial. She also had the opportunity to join a group for newly diagnosed/minimally disabled M.S. persons that was sponsored by her local Multiple Sclerosis Society. She found the Patients' Services Division of the Society particularly helpful. There were two other teens in the group, and they seemed to help each other.

The process of acceptance was, in fact, under way for Gloria before she was even fully aware of it. Once she verbalized the need for change, she was beginning to adjust and adapt her life-style. A few meetings later, she shared her new concept with the group. She explained to them that "I have learned this week to stretch an elastic around me with no rigid boundary between me and my symptoms. The key to stretching is giving up the importance of what everyone else thinks. I was not even disturbed this week when I caught a glimpse of my limp in a store window. I am now stretching and accepting. No one was there to judge."

Old ways of assessing oneself are replaced by new, more realistic ways in the adapting/adjusting stage. Perspective broadens as the M.S. person begins to reemerge into society. He is better able to see himself with talents and strengths that are not connected to his illness. M.S. becomes only a part of a person's life—not the whole of it. It shrinks in importance with time. Though the symptoms are always present, the M.S. person sees adapting to the symptoms as secondary to meeting all other goals for life's enrichment.

Gloria's parents did help her immeasurably. They led her to a therapist who understood both adolescents and M.S. Her parents did not get stuck in advancing headlong to do as they wanted—namely, continue to attempt to answer all of Gloria's needs themselves as they had done when she was younger. Her father adds, "Though we were often tempted, we didn't go the other way either. We didn't ever throw up our hands and leave her free to exert her own authority. If we had, she could have remained in her room forever," he concludes. Instead, her parents allowed her to develop her own independent relationship with her therapist and members of her M.S. support group.

In addition, a teen's uncertainty about body-image can contribute to a denial of the potential body harm that accident, injury, or illness may bring. Parents shake their heads at a younger person's risk-taking behavior, whether it be fast driving, aggressive athletics, or substance abuse, and wonder at how "he acts as if nothing can hurt him." They are acknowledging a fantasy of invulnerability that adolescents adopt to cover over their anxious concerns about their bodies and, more fundamentally, death and finitude. When illness cracks open the fragile shell of denial and fantasy, anxiety and a deeper sense of helplessness and hopelessness emerge.

"After I imagined the worst possible fate for myself," Jean relates, "I was terrified and I wanted my mother near to hold me. I felt as if I were four or five. I remembered how good I felt when I got out of the bath and she wrapped a towel around me and powdered me with talcum. I was so safe then, and now something terrible was happening to me. It didn't seem fair. I wanted my mother to fix it."

Although not all teenagers are as articulate as Jean, most young people are conscious of their yearning for comfort and rescue in the face of unfavorable events. They are close enough to their childhoods to still hope for a parental act of saving grace. They are not yet old enough to have transferred their expectations for healing onto doctors or science. The inability of parents to be all powerful protectors is a difficult fact for many of them to accept.

Says Jean's mother, "I never felt worse than when Jean's diagnosis was made. My sorrow for her was accompanied by a tremendous sense of guilt. My husband and I felt that we had missed all the early signs, dismissing them as 'normal clumsiness,' although the doctors said there was absolutely no way we could have known otherwise.

"But the deeper guilt was for not protecting our child, failing to keep her from harm. We know it isn't rational, but I think it's an emotion that is part of what makes parent-love. Maybe we have a biological need to care for our young. Whatever the reason, I know that when we believe that we fail in that task, we suffer and are, in some way, ashamed of ourselves."

Soon Jean also felt guilty, believing her illness was a burden on her parents. She saw their unhappiness and took on the responsibility for it. She thought her illness deprived them of the normal satisfaction she assumed they took in their family life. She also became quite upset that the progression of her M.S. might leave her parents taking care of her well after the time she should have been on her own and they would have been enjoying their years without responsibility for children. She even felt guilty when she was concerned with her health and her own future.

Jean's condition following her diagnosis remained stable. There were times when she walked unsteadily and occasionally had dizzy spells and some fatigue, but in general she functioned pretty much as she had before. Still, her life had changed, as Jean points out.

"Both my parents were always asking how I was, if I felt okay, if there was anything they could do for me. During this time, I was attending school and actually living quite normally. I think I just shoved my anxiety about my M.S. to the back of my head. My parents began to annoy me. It was like they kept harping on what I didn't want to think about. I could understand their concern, but I wanted them to stop.

"They also became uptight about my dating and curfews and stuff like that," Jean continues. "If I was going out with someone, they asked more questions than they ever had before. I think they thought I was more fragile or would be taken advantage of because of my condition. In fact, the people who treated me most differently were my parents, not my friends."

Because the development of identity for a teen re-
volves around peer contact, the end result is the spending of less time at home and more time involved with
friends. Parents, especially parents of an M.S. teen,
must encourage this interaction, which is necessary for
the development of an increased social confidence.
Similarly, when teens become involved with clothes and
peer influences on taste of wardrobes, it is even more
important for parents to encourage this sense of feeling
attractive and being accepted by friends. The ability to
make decisions about taste in clothes, friends, and
activities all encourages independent thinking, so natural for other teens and so essential for the M.S. person.

Jean's mother points out what was going on for her
husband and her. "We felt so guilty about our failure to
protect Jean that perhaps we overreacted by setting too
many limits on her. We watched closely over her, trying
to keep away any misfortune. We attempted to cope with
our own inability to control either our anxiety or the
disease. Looking back, I think we could have been more
relaxed about her social life, but I think she now
understands why we acted as we did."

Jean also was aware of her increased dependence upon
her parents. When she thought they were exerting too
much control over her life, she became very critical of
them. When they reacted with anger, she felt even more
justified in her rejection of their concern. Although what
went on between Jean and her parents is normal enough
for teenagers, some of the vehemence in their conflicts
was generated by the ambivalence both parties felt about
dependency issues highlighted by Jean's illness. The
guilt each party feels over a variety of different issues
intensifies the friction and can create situations that all
regret.

Though desires for independence and some autonomy

for developing one's plans and philosophy of life separate from one's parents constitute an important developmental phase in all teens, for the M.S. teenager it is sometimes more essential to reach out to other adults at school or in the community. To have a confidante or mentor in the form of a teacher or the parent of a friend can often alleviate the guilt and dependency issues that occur in the home.

When Jean first began to confide in her friend Sue's mother, her own parents began to feel insulted and snubbed. "We felt such love and responsibility for her," her mother admits, "that we found ourselves wishing she'd act as if she appreciated our presence. Seeking out another parent made us feel we were being snubbed." Yet the ability to consult another adult often lessens the emotional conflicts that exist at home. The home issues can often be put in perspective by an uninvolved yet caring adult. Jean's mother soon became less insulted and more relieved to find that Sue's mother was sharing the awesome responsibility of presenting the adult view to Jean. "Jean began to put my comments in perspective after airing them with Sue's mother, and I was grateful."

Sometimes, however, young people seem to resign rather than continue to fight and accept a role of greater dependency than their condition or need warrants. Emotions can run very high and we advise parents and young people to seek counseling if the struggle seems more intense than what one expects or wants. The issues here—parental guilt and adolescent fears of loss or control and autonomy—are important to confront in a helpful way.

In addition to the psychological dynamics we have described here, there are additional sources of stress present in families with an adolescent or young adult sick at home. Parents may have to modify career goals in light of the need for extended time to care for their child, or they may have to alter plans for vacations and leisure activities. There may well be increased financial burden due to the cost of medical and support services, housing modifications, various therapies, and so on. Parents may well have to spend a lot of time and effort getting proper medical care and follow-through for their youngster as well as make sure any physical impairment does not deprive the child of any educational opportunities.

Strained family relationships, however, make other stresses more difficult to cope with. Parents may feel resentful about the increased time and financial commitment that a sick child requires and may direct their anger at that young person. On the other hand, it is not unusual for parents to vent their frustrations on each other. Unfortunately, just when the family needs strong and mutually supportive parents, the worry and anxiety over the illness may begin to break down the marital relationship. The adolescent with M.S. may feel responsible for any family disharmony or conflict. They blame themselves for parental inadequacies.

Andy was diagnosed with multiple sclerosis when he was seventeen. A junior in high school, he was an average student and anticipated attending college and then entering his father's construction business. Although possessed of fine athletic abilities, he did not participate in sports; instead, with a friend, he operated an odd-jobs business—painting, hauling trash, cleaning cellars, and so on. As his parents said, he was a "good kid" with a normal and active social life that included occasional dating and beer drinking with his buddies.

"Andy's initial symptoms," Elaine, Andy's mother, says, "were excessive fatigue, visual disturbances, and

some coordination loss. Initially, we thought mononucleosis to be a possibility, but tests revealed no evidence
of that illness. After several near automobile accidents
we feared that drug or alcohol abuse was involved, and
we had several loud arguments where Andy denied our
accusations. Of course, we feel terrible about those
fights now. His teachers and guidance counselor also
became concerned as Andy's performance dropped off.
Finally, friends prevailed on us to bring Andy to a
therapist to see what his emotional problems were.

"Andy went along with the visits but no one could
identify any particular reasons why he was feeling the
way he did. We were about to chalk everything up to
normal adolescent turmoil when the therapist suggested
some educational and personality testing to see whether
there might be sources of stress or school difficulties that
we weren't picking up.

"Fortunately, the psychologists who did the testing
were connected with a neurological group and had
experience working with individuals with M.S. After
Andy described his symptoms, just on a hunch one of
them suggested a neurological appointment. After several months of tests and examinations, multiple sclerosis
was given as a probable diagnosis.

"My husband and I were stunned. We felt such deep
pain for Andy. What can be worse than the pain a parent
feels for a child's misfortune? But Andy was quiet. He
didn't cry. He didn't act scared. He told us not to worry.
He'd be okay. No problem is what he said.

"And then Andy changed. He fought with his younger
sister, whom he'd always treated so well. He argued with
us about everything. Curfews meant nothing to him.
He'd stay out late and give us any excuse. He lied. His
schoolwork plummeted. B's turned to C's and soon to

failures. We begged him to go for counseling, to listen to his doctors. He refused. He'd live for now, he said, he didn't know what the future would be, so why bother living for that. Grades didn't mean anything. He said that before his body fell apart he wanted to make sure he got a lot of use out of it.

"He was running full throttle. We were in despair. No matter how often we told him that the doctors had been pretty optimistic about the course of his illness, he kept running. He was looking for trouble and trouble was looking for him. He was so afraid and we felt helpless. We tried being angry, we tried being calm. We set limits, we gave him full rein. We followed through with consequences, we offered rewards. Whatever therapists, friends, or books suggested, we tried. And still our son was bent, it seemed, on his own destruction. What multiple sclerosis might do to him could be no worse than what he was inflicting upon himself.

"Finally, we found a therapist who helped us focus on ourselves. In our attempts to reach out to Andy we had neglected to give the rest of us the nurturing we needed. Our daughter, Alexis, felt most neglected. And what my husband and I did to each other with all our blaming and worrying was terrible. In our understandable obsession with Andy's out of control reaction, we had put our entire family in jeopardy, including the support he would need when he slowed down.

"And one day he did. Not in the way we would wish, but it was a first step. He was impatient with a school bus that stopped in front of him and he pulled out to pass, almost hitting a group of children crossing the street. A police officer saw it all and actually arrested him for reckless endangerment. As an alternative to a court appearance, he entered a court-sponsored counseling program where for the first time he began to see the potential consequences of his behavior on others, if not on himself.

"The path from that near tragedy to coming to terms with the diagnosis of multiple sclerosis was a long and difficult one. But with our support, a helpful therapist who had a terrific relationship with Andy, and Andy's courage, he made it. He took the rest of the year off from school and spent some time just relaxing. The friends from whom he had pulled away stuck by him and he even got a girlfriend. I think she did more to help him get back his physical confidence than anyone else.

"Looking back," Elaine sums up, "I don't know if we could have done anything different with Andy. I suppose he had to work out his demons his own way; I'm just happy he made it without hurting himself or anyone else. I'm so glad we found our therapist, who helped us stop hurting each other and helped keep our guilt and shame at bay. We do let each other know how much we care and we do stop to smell the roses a little more often. Some of the things Andy said about life's shortness in his fear and panic have a great deal of truth in them and we acknowledge that. It's hard to say anything good could come from something like multiple sclerosis, but we are a stronger and better family now."

Siblings may also be in emotional turmoil. "I know that Jean's brother and sister felt terrible and afraid about Jean's M.S.," Jean's mother explains. "We let the doctors tell them they had nothing to fear about themselves getting M.S., and they were relieved. But they continued, of course, to feel badly about Jean.

"As time passed, however, and we had to change or cancel family outings or cut down on vacation plans, they became very annoyed. They were reluctant to express it, because they thought they were mean to have such thoughts. They didn't tell us what they were thinking and they didn't get angry at Jean, so they began to fight more frequently with each other and became more irritable with friends. When Jean's father and I also began to argue more, the younger ones began to do a little more poorly in school. Fortunately we sought counseling before the situation deteriorated any further."

The therapist helped Jean's parents cope with their feelings of loss—of Jean's good health, of their ability to protect their children from all harm, of their fantasies and expectations for their family and their own future together as a couple, of smoothly coping with expected family crises, of their idea of "the good life," which somehow excluded illness, accident, or the unexpected.

The entire family got a chance to talk openly about their feelings. They discovered that many of the thoughts and emotions they felt were theirs alone were also shared by others. Much of the tension they experienced was a result of failing to acknowledge to each other their secret thoughts, of which they were ashamed and about which they believed they would be judged.

It was helpful to Jean's siblings to hear that she sometimes resented their good health and felt bad when she did. Jean found it useful to know that her siblings sometimes stayed away from her because they felt guilty about the anger they had toward her for changing their lives. The therapist pointed out that anger was an entirely appropriate response, but it was better directed at the M.S. and the family's altered circumstances than toward each other.

When members of a family attempt to keep their feelings secret from one another, there is a tendency for some kind of dysfunctional behavior to emerge. It may be expressed as anger to justify the lack of sharing, distancing to keep the experience of guilt and shame at bay, or overdependence and overprotectiveness to "make up" for "bad" feelings. A family that treats chronic illness and the complex psychological dynamics that surround it as something not to be discussed becomes a confusing dance of frightened individuals stumbling, grabbing, or avoiding each other in the dark. The truth about what people feel, once revealed, is rarely as dangerous as what is imagined.

❧ 10 ❧

Staying as Healthy as Possible

THERE IS NO QUESTION that the day-to-day struggle to cope with multiple sclerosis can be exhausting. One often despairs that the course of the illness can ever be stilled or any losses of strength or function regained. The attempt to stay even—physically, mentally, or emotionally—with a chronic disease may seem noble, yet it seems so futile.

Yet many fear that not struggling is surrendering. Some people suggest, for example, "doing battle" with an illness to overcome it. They see the illness as an enemy within the body, an alien attacker. Others believe that living as if the disability does not exist is the best policy. Both these approaches seem flawed to us. The first creates an unnecessary antagonism between different aspects of oneself. The second denies the reality of both the disease and the human capacity for healing.

Attitude

It is possible to foster attitudes and take actions that make living with multiple sclerosis easier and may, in the long run, influence its progression and outcomes. The first step in this middle way between struggle and surrender is to recognize that a disease is *not* a judgment or a punishment. Multiple sclerosis is something that happens to a person because of a variety of factors, known and unknown. There is no blame.

A second step is to realize that a person is neither all-powerful nor helpless to cope with her illness. She *can* live so that her illness affects, but does *not* control, her life. An individual *is* responsible for defining and choosing what the illness means for her.

Does my having M.S. mean I am a victim, doomed to suffer the ravages of an illness that will destroy me and whom and what I love? Or is my misfortune a challenge to meet difficulty with some measure of grace, courage, and compassion for myself and others? How one answers this question is more important than any symptoms or disability a disease may bring.

A third step is to establish a relationship with one's M.S. Unwanted as it may be, multiple sclerosis is a lifelong partner, for better or for worse, in sickness and in health. To view it as an enemy or to ignore its presence does not, unfortunately, make it disappear. One must get to know it, live with it, come to terms with it.

Of course, this does not mean that M.S. is your friend. Rather, one must accept it as an unwelcome companion on a long journey. Acquaint yourself with its moods, departures, and returns. Keep a wary eye upon it; know when to rest, to push, to struggle, and to compromise.

And unlike with a friend, rejoice at its retreats and regret its arrivals.

Acknowledging the reality of the effects of M.S. upon your life and its potential impact upon your future is a crucial fourth step. It would be wise, for example, to consider how one's employment might be disrupted by M.S. and to investigate alternative career paths. Because you may lose the opportunity to obtain disability insurance, preparations for financial security must be made.

Some people feel overwhelmed, not so much by the immediate problem as by the possible or long-term implications of M.S. for themselves and their families. It takes great courage to face these issues squarely, but one must do so. It is worthwhile to undergo the anxiety involved in dealing with these practical matters, rather than put them off. Hoping that bad things will go away does not make them disappear.

The next step is to imagine the kind of future you want for yourself. Do you want to be physically, emotionally, and mentally healthy? To move with grace, mobility, and assurance? To function effectively at work and at home? To develop and maintain satisfying relationships with family and friends? To meet and cope with exacerbations in a calm and productive way? These are challenges and goals to be reached for, not tests to be failed or passed.

A person may not attain what he aims for. Yet the stretch toward what he wants reinforces and nourishes a self-pride that is a source of enormous confidence, determination, and strength. A life based upon what one aspires to is of a different grain than one that flounders around what a person wants to avoid.

The path of life for a person with multiple sclerosis does not differ fundamentally from anyone else's. There is an old tale about a man who complains about his lot in life. An angel shows him a tree on which knapsacks hang from every limb. The angel invites the man to look inside each bundle and choose which he wants. After gazing into all of them, the man decides to keep his own. The knapsacks contain other men's troubles.

Managing Stress

In imagining the life you want for yourself, it is important to be aware of how stress affects your body. Stress, of course, is something each person experiences in life. Many people enjoy a certain amount of stress and find it pushes them toward greater risk or achievement. For other people, smaller amounts of stress can be quite harmful. For most people, the pressure of chronic, unwanted stress is debilitating.

It is common for people with M.S. to find that stress causes a temporary worsening of their symptoms. It can increase both the severity and the frequency of exacerbations. When a person is calm, rested, and relaxed, the physical organism can cope with life events effectively, but during times of anxiety and tension, symptoms may flare up.

Louise, the psychiatrist, reports that under stress her legs don't work as well. "When I stand to greet a new patient, I'm occasionally embarrassed by how long it takes me to rise and balance. Sometimes, as I begin to shake hands, I find I have to balance myself with my other hand. Also, when I'm feeling this way, my tongue seems to stumble a bit and my speech worsens." Though these responses are temporary and nonprogressive, they are frustrating.

Louise decided to ameliorate the impact of stress by learning and using simple methods of relaxation. When she practiced these techniques, flare-ups of the M.S. lessened. In addition, the complications of leg problems, muscle weakness, and loss of fluency in speech that had previously occurred on stressful days almost disappeared. Louise felt better and more in control.

Relaxation

When existing tension makes it harder to cope with new difficulties, short relaxation exercises can break the stress cycle and help body parts to relax and reduce much of the physical, emotional, and mental strain that accompanies M.S. The following simple exercises are easy to do in your home.

1. From a standing or sitting position, stretch your arms as high as you can reach. Then bend your body from the waist and let your arms hang in front of you. Repeat this exercise ten times, without strain, reaching and stretching each time.
2. Pull your shoulders back and rotate them forward and back five times. Do a few gentle head rolls at the end.
3. Close your eyes, slowly inhale and exhale, allowing your abdomen to rise as air enters. Breathe in and out, relaxing completely.

This prepares you to be relaxed and alert for the relaxation exercise that follows. Try these exercises at the same time each day in a quiet environment. Some kinds of music may be an aid to exercise.

The following method of relaxation has been used in many cultures throughout history. The background of the technique and its documented effectiveness may be found in *The Relaxation Response* by Herbert Benson, M.D., published by Avon Books.

MEDITATION

The following meditation exercise is taken from *Maximizing Your Health*, edited by Robert Buxbaum, M.D., and Debra Frankel, M.S., O.T.R., published by the Massachusetts chapter of the National Multiple Sclerosis Society, 400-1 Totten Pond Road, Waltham, MA 02154. This is an excellent program of graded exercise and meditation for people with multiple sclerosis. We recommend it to all.

1. Depending on your preference and physical condition, sit either on a chair or on cushions on the floor or in bed. Keep your back comfortably straight so that you can breathe naturally; let your eyes close gently.

2. Draw your attention inward and begin to center your attention on your breathing. Without trying to breathe more deeply or control your breath in any way, feel how the abdomen expands and contracts like a balloon as you inhale and exhale. Now relax your muscles as best you can, starting at your feet and working toward your head. Breathe in and then out; let go of any tension in your feet. Move up to your ankles, again letting tension go as you exhale. In this way, work up your body, relaxing your lower legs, thighs, buttocks, chest, back, shoulders, neck, upper arms, lower arms, hands, and then your face and scalp.

3. Continue to focus your attention on your breathing, centering on the contraction and expansion of your abdomen. On each exhale, silently repeat a word or phrase of your choice. It can be "relax," "peace," "one," a short prayer, or an affirmation such as "better and better"

or "stronger and stronger." Don't change from one word to another. Make a choice and stick with it. The word or phrase serves as a further focus for your concentration, allowing you to let go of the many stressful thoughts about the past or future that create tension.

4. Keep a passive attitude. It is natural for thoughts to enter your mind and for your concentration to wander. You will be amazed at how busy your mind is! Identify the drift of the mind and just let it go. You can return to your thoughts later. Meanwhile, return to the breathing and the repetition of your word or phrase. In time, it will become easier to concentrate.

Continue the meditation for ten minutes, longer if you can. At the end, sit quietly for a minute or two with your eyes closed. Begin to think of the exercises you will do; imagine yourself doing them to the very best of your ability. Then let your eyes open gradually; sit for another moment before you begin your daily routine.

The goal of these exercises is not to eliminate stress. To most of us, that would mean eliminating the living process. Many people thrive on stress. Without it life would be boring. Negative stress can, however, trigger exacerbations as well as affect our digestive systems, heartbeat, and blood pressure. Learning how to disengage from stressful thoughts and feelings through calming meditation is essential to control the complications of chronic illness.

PHYSICAL EXERCISE

Walking, swimming, and other regular physical exercise are helpful ways of reducing the effects of stress. The authors of *Maximizing Your Health* point out that much of the body and organ systems are unaffected by M.S. Although the specific benefits of exercise for people with

M.S. are not known, there is little doubt that maximizing overall health contributes to resistance to disease, increased energy, and a greater feeling of well-being.

The exercise program described in *Maximizing Your Health* emphasizes improving strength, flexibility, and endurance for individuals. What is particularly unique about this book is its exercise levels for people with different ambulatory abilities:

Level A—independent;

Level B—independent with assistance of crutch, cane, or walker;

Level C—wheelchair mobile.

The program is flexible so that individuals who are Level A in some exercises may function at Level B or Level C in other exercises. We strongly recommend this book.

Diet

There is no diet capable of healing M.S. or designed strictly for people with M.S. Diet and nutrition are, however, important to overall health. The healthiest diet for most people is also the optimal way for those with M.S. to eat.

No one diet, of course, is ideal for all. Nevertheless, dietary guidelines have been established for healthy Americans to use as a basis for food selection. A well-balanced diet includes portions from the major food groups, including fruits and vegetables, whole grain or enriched breads, cereals, dairy products, and protein foods such as fish, poultry, legumes, meat, or eggs.

Other worthwhile hints for healthy eating include maintaining a normal weight for your frame, which is particularly important for more inactive and less mobile people with M.S., as well as avoiding too much fat and eating food with adequate starch and fiber. Too much sugar, salt, and alcohol should be avoided.

The following are suggestions for reducing fat in the diet:

Limit consumption of cream, butter, hydrogenated margarine or shortening, and products made with these;

Use low-fat or skim milk;

Limit the consumption of fatty meats and cheese;

Avoid frying;

Use lean meats, poultry, fish, dried peas or beans, and tofu as protein sources.

To improve eating habits, it is important to eat slowly, prepare smaller portions, and avoid tempting "seconds."

A word about alcohol: Alcohol should be used prudently by individuals with M.S. It is a central nervous system depressant and individuals with balance and coordination problems are very likely to be adversely affected by it. The possibility of accident or injury is increased by its excessive use. Also, problems with incontinence or urgency to urinate are likely to be exacerbated by alcohol. If you wish to drink, do so slowly and carefully follow these guidelines for safe drinking:

Know that you may choose not to drink and can say "no" to alcoholic beverages for any reason;

Don't drink and drive;

Don't drink alone;

If you are a woman, realize that alcohol will have a greater effect on you even if you weigh the same as a man;

Drink slowly and avoid gulping a drink—alcohol is a drug;

Don't make drinking the main focus of your social event;

Recognize that the use of alcohol for purposes of coping with problems is a high-risk behavior (if you feel you are having a problem, consult someone);

If you are depressed, avoid alcohol; it is a depressant.

We have presented a prescription for maintaining as good health as possible—a positive and realistic attitude, effectively coping with stress using methods of relaxation and meditation, a regular program of exercise, and a low-fat diet. No one can guarantee that the result will be a decrease in frequency and severity of exacerbations, but can a person with M.S. cure her disease by following medical, nutritional, or spiritual instruction of any kind? Unfortunately the answer at this time is still no.

It is true, however, that how people perceive their potential for effective living can influence their future behavior and health. An individual with a strong positive attitude, armed with the necessary medical information and guidance, can have a say in the quality of his life. The fact of illness provides some limits on what is possible; it does not limit the attitude one takes toward one's self and one's life.

Healing, health, wealth, and wholeness all come from the same root word. They originally applied more to spiritual attitude and state of mind than to physical function. A man enfeebled by age, injury, or even disease could nonetheless be said to be healthy, wealthy, and wise if he treated others with kindness and respect and fulfilled his obligations as well as he was able. Conversely, a man of cruelty, whatever his physical well-being, would be regarded as more animal than person, someone with a sickness of the soul in need of healing. A chronic illness of the body need not become a disease of spirit and mind. Each person makes a choice.

❖ 11 ❖

Practical
Considerations

Recreation and Travel

ONE OF THE MOST frustrating aspects of chronic illness or disability is the effect it has on leisure-time activities. Just when a person would benefit most from the relaxation, enjoyment, and socialization that come from recreation, he is limited in what he can do. It is important, however, despite whatever limitations may exist, to maintain existing or find new interests.

Although it is understandable that a person may be discouraged from or inhibited in associating with old friends or in trying out new partners, it is wise to do so. Some multiple sclerosis chapters sponsor summer programs for people with M.S. to facilitate this necessary interaction. An example is the family week at a summer camp that the Massachusetts M.S. Chapter offers in New Hampshire each year.

There is also a network of horseback riding programs for the physically challenged. Many people with M.S.

find that riding builds back abdominal muscles, strengthens weak legs, and is a terrific source of self-confidence.

There are also groups throughout the country that provide instruction and modified equipment for skiing, bicycling, and just about every other sport. Marathon spectators have become accustomed to seeing competitors on crutches or in wheelchairs arriving at the finish line. For the sports and exercise enthusiast with multiple sclerosis, much is available.

Travel for a person with M.S. has never been easier. Although it is never simple—you must take the time to check out what is available and from whom—you will find that many airlines, airports, trains, and car rental companies offer services to make your journey more comfortable and, indeed, possible. There are also increasing numbers of books, newsletters, and organizations that provide information about the best sites to visit, restaurants, accommodations, shopping areas, and means of transportation for people with limited mobility.

It is also wise to make sure that you will have access to any personal care or medical equipment or services you may need when you travel. Often, purchasing supplies prior to departure will take care of potential problems. In general, writing or calling ahead for what you need to know to enjoy your travel experiences is good advice. Also, there may be people you know with some disability who have traveled and can offer some thought about what works and what doesn't, precautions to take, and good bets for enjoyment.

Housing

Many people with multiple sclerosis find that some modification of their home helps make daily life more convenient, comfortable, and safe. The addition of a ramp or lift for a wheelchair helps make it easier to get outside. For some individuals, grab bars or safety mats in the shower make a difference. For others, remodeling an existing bathroom is often necessary for additional convenience, and moving a laundry room to the same floor as the bedrooms can conserve energy and add to efficiency.

There are many products on the market to help people work faucets, open doors, and operate appliances. Local M.S. chapters as well as many other organizations for the physically challenged can help you identify and obtain the resources you need, including architects and contractors who can modify your living space to meet your needs.

Some people may have to change location. Transportation may be a problem, there may be resistance on the part of the landlord to making structural changes, or stairs may be too difficult to negotiate. Again, local M.S. chapters, hospital social workers, community agencies, and clergy can help people locate appropriate housing. For individuals who live alone, one solution may be cooperative living arrangements with other people. Whatever the circumstances, the extended family is obliged, we believe, to help create an enjoyable and suitable living situation.

Transportation and Access

Getting around as much as possible with a minimum of inconvenience is the goal of all people with a physical disability. In the past, the major obstacle to maximizing one's mobility has been the architectural barriers to full access to public and private facilities, including side-walks, stairways, offices, and stores.

A second roadblock to going where one wants to go has been a lack of accessible public transportation and affordable adapted vehicles. Many of these difficulties are being eliminated, although often at too slow a pace, through force of law, public support, and awakened and aggressive consumer demand. But there are still too many unnecessary barriers of all kinds that thwart the most determined person in a wheelchair.

Wheelchairs are lighter now and some are made especially for transportation in a car trunk or station wagon. More people than ever before drive vehicles with adaptive equipment and as the ease of use rises, the cost for such equipment will drop. A book from the American Automobile Association, *The Handicapped Driver's Mobility Guide*, describes and lists laws, adaptive equipment and vehicles, and financing sources available for the physically challenged driver.

Clinical Resources

The financial costs of a chronic illness can be substantial, if not staggering. Medical care, rehabilitation, ambulatory and adaptive equipment, home modification and reconstruction, personal care, and the loss of income from a change in employment all contribute to the huge burden felt by the individual and his family. It can happen that the money saved toward a child's college education must be redirected to pay the debts incurred by a parent's illness; the ill parent's own sense of satisfaction and self-worth become defined by how many payments can be made for medical services past due.

Local M.S. chapters can help people with multiple sclerosis identify existing and potential resources they may have or be able to use to meet the financial needs associated with their illness. These include: private health and disability insurance; federal and state programs such as Social Security disability, Medicare, or supplemental security income benefits and Veterans Administration benefits; and state programs, particularly for vocational rehabilitation. It is not easy to go through the process of finding out what you are entitled to and how to go about getting it. It can be frustrating and even heartbreaking. We suggest you develop a good relationship with someone in your local M.S. chapter's Patients' Services Division, or a local community social service agency that can help you navigate through these sometimes difficult shoals.

Just as one plans for retirement or meeting the expense of college tuition, it is helpful to do realistic financial planning for the potential consequences of chronic illness and disability. Good planning begins with knowing what your current resources are, setting some goals, and, especially with multiple sclerosis, anticipating the unexpected. If one partner cannot work as fully as before, can the other partner make up the difference? Is disability insurance, assuming one has it, sufficient to meet needs? Is it wiser to be financially conservative and build assets or use money now for pleasures that may be more difficult to enjoy if the illness progresses? Are there expenses that could be eliminated now to help build equity and cash reserve? These are not easy questions, but they can be very useful in staving off a catastrophic financial situation down the line. Forewarned is to be forearmed.

There is no easy or permanent solution to the problem

of money. It may seem unfair that those who have the greatest need may have the fewest resources to meet that need. There is no doubt that the burden is upon you and your family to make contingency plans and meet the financial obligations that result from chronic illness. Your options may be few; your choices hard. Nevertheless, you can put yourself in a better position by sound record keeping, short- and long-term planning, and realistic goals.

Advocacy and Rights

Having an illness such as multiple sclerosis for many people means having to come to terms with the psychological, social, and political realities of physical disability. Whether one employs the word "handicapped" or not, the fact is that if your mobility is limited or your capacity for full-functioning impaired, you are entitled to certain rights and protections under the law. It is your right to take full advantage of the law to secure greater access to your city or town, more employment and educational opportunities, workplaces modified for your needs, and financial benefits for better medical care and housing.

It is easy to simply put up with obstacles to full access and overlook them as inconveniences you must learn to tolerate, but it would be wrong to do so. They are unnecessary and, perhaps, unlawful chains that prevent you from fulfilling your potential.

One young woman with multiple sclerosis asked her college professor if she could use a tape recorder to record his lectures and review them at home. Susan had weakness and tremors in her hand and some visual problems. He refused her request. She accepted his refusal, but when Susan mentioned the event to a group of people with M.S., they were outraged. Apart from the professor's lack of sensitivity to her needs, they knew that his refusal to help her compensate for her disability was in violation of state and federal law. They encouraged Susan to return to class and let him know that she would report the incident to the school administration and the M.S. Society. When she told him that, he naturally relented.

Susan is typically nonassertive, and she was unwilling to pursue the matter legally. But her confrontation with her professor was a significant step. Since then, she has become much more aggressive in ensuring that people know of and respect her illness.

There is one problem that has kept people with chronic illnesses and disability from achieving all the rights to which they are entitled and all the benefits that full participation and access would give them. It is the failure to identify with others who may have similar, but not identical, needs. People with multiple sclerosis need to realize that many of the difficulties they have are obstacles faced by other physically challenged individuals. They also have problems with housing, transportation, insurance, Social Security, discrimination, and employment. Joining with others is often the most effective way to create the political power necessary to effect change.

In addition, people with chronic illness and disability must deal with the day-to-day problems of health and coping. It is up to family members to take the lead in individual and group advocacy, including legal action when necessary, to ensure individuals their rights and fair benefits. Local chapters of the M.S. Society and other support and advocacy groups can help people find lawyers and legal-aid groups interested in and sympathetic to obtaining the rights of disabled people. Asserting oneself is not easy, but many times it is the only way to get what you need, want, and deserve.

The National Multiple Sclerosis Society

Throughout this book we have mentioned the National Multiple Sclerosis Society as an effective organization working on behalf of people with multiple sclerosis, their families, health-care professionals, and the many scientists and others engaged in research for treating and curing this unfortunate disease. Any person with M.S. and his or her family ought to contact their local chapter in order to learn more about the organization and its many services.

Many chapters offer a variety of programs, such as:

Education, including professional seminars, in-service training programs, public education, courses, and informational meetings for newly diagnosed individuals and their families;

Self-help support groups, including telephone networks;

Research, which is partially funded by local chapters and the National Society;

Newsletters to keep people up to date with latest research findings, new resources for living and coping with M.S., educational meetings, and more;

Counseling services, including peer, individual, family, and group counseling;

Information and referral services, including a number of informational pamphlets and a list of additional reading materials (some chapters have lending libraries);

Advocacy services on behalf of people with M.S. to help them obtain the right to equal access, equal opportunity, and good and necessary health care;

And additional special services, such as procuring medical or therapeutic equipment, emergency transportation, home-care visits.

Of course, not all chapters provide all services, nor are they able to provide many services for particular individuals over the long term, but they are the first place to turn for correct information about M.S. and resources for coping with it. A list of local chapters of the Multiple Sclerosis Society and the National Multiple Sclerosis Society is included at the end of this book, as well as a list of pamphlets available from the National Society.

As we said at the beginning of the book, life is painful. But it can be sweet and filled with love. What we owe ourselves and each other is compassion for the struggle we each make to live our lives as best we can. And, of course, this is true for all, regardless of our physical condition, mental abilities, or emotional state.

❖ 12 ❖

The Biological Bases of M.S.: Implications for Research and Treatment

THE PURPOSE OF THIS CHAPTER is to better inform M.S. patients and their families on the significance of what you may hear or read. It is hard enough for experts in the field of M.S. to judge claims in the news media or in scientific articles; it is even harder for the layman.

We cannot cover everything that is currently known about multiple sclerosis, so here we'll just try to simplify the complex medical material so that the average person can understand, in general, what the current "state of the art" of M.S. research and therapy is today. Obviously, anything can change tomorrow—and may even change before the written word comes off the press.

Another goal is to allow you to appreciate the uniqueness of each individual with M.S. Hopefully you have begun to appreciate where your case is different from all others and where it fits into the big picture of *individualized* patient management.

Clinical Events and Pathological Correlations

Most of the common symptoms and signs of multiple sclerosis may be correlated with particular findings in the central nervous system. For example, impaired vision in one eye may be associated with findings of optic neuritis. Attacks of double vision may be associated with loss of myelin around nerve pathways in the brain stem, involving areas that control coordination of eye movements. Weakness or numbness in the legs may be related to findings of myelin loss in a patchy fashion throughout the spinal cord or in some cases at a single level of the cord. Different parts of the nervous system are involved in different individuals and at different times in the same individual. There is a tendency for selective areas to be picked out in some M.S. patients, such as motor pathways to legs, coordination centers, or visual apparatus.

When tissues are examined, either grossly or microscopically, the areas of myelin loss stand out as somewhat gelatinous, discolored areas. They tend to congregate mainly around the chambers of the brain known as the ventricles and also around veins in the brain or spinal cord.

Usually, a neurologist can pinpoint where demyelination has occurred by examining the patient and localizing the findings to specific areas of the central nervous system. This can be done with a relatively simple office or outpatient examination.

The diagnosis can be confirmed beyond any doubt

with noninvasive testing such as evoked responses that test visual, brain stem auditory, or somatosensory pathways through the spinal cord. These tests, which are harmless to the patient, may demonstrate additional areas of involvement not defined by medical history or neurological examination alone.

A spinal tap (lumbar puncture, or L.P.), using a local anesthetic such as Xylocaine, is performed, usually with minimal discomfort. The laboratory technician looks for cellular reaction in the spinal fluid and checks for the kinds of protein changes that are common in M.S. The laboratory can measure levels of myelin basic protein, oligoclonal band patterns in the protein, and alterations of the immune proteins manifest by elevated levels of IgG or gamma globulin. IgG is an immune globulin which is sometimes elevated in persons with M.S. The details are not necessary for you to know; but in general, there are relatively specific protein changes suggestive of M.S. that are present during attacks or in the progressive state; however, these are not present in every single case.

In addition, a CAT scan with extra doses of contrast material, or, better yet, Magnetic Resonance Imaging, will produce pictures of the brain or spinal cord and show the extent of demyelinated areas in many, but not all, cases.

Possible Causes of M.S.

Currently the two most popular theories of causation are the infectious or viral theory and the autoimmune theory. In simple terms, there is evidence to suggest that a slow-acting virus acquired many years ago, possibly prior to age fifteen, may trigger a series of slow reactions that lead to the ultimate formation of antibodies. One may find antibodies against specific viruses which affect the central nervous system. In addition, components in the brain may react to the antibody by making excessive amounts of myelin basic protein. Finally, antibodies may react against chemicals in the central nervous system, thereby attacking the patient's proteins instead of the foreign viral agent.

Current theories hold that antibodies produced in the body to fight a foreign substance or foreign virus instead attack substances known as amino acids that "look like" the invader. Because of problems in its formation, the antibody cannot distinguish one amino acid from the other. What then happens is the antibodies turn against the patient's own myelin and body proteins when they should have reacted only against the foreign substance.

This immune reaction triggers exacerbations of M.S. Certain individuals are more predisposed genetically to the disease if they have susceptible genes in their makeup. The most susceptible genes are known as the HLA-DR2 type. In research programs, scientists can identify these susceptible genes.

Other predisposing factors have been learned from epidemiological studies of different ethnic groups in different parts of the world. Those that live in northern latitudes are more predisposed with the possible exception of the Japanese. Those who live closer to the equator are less predisposed. If you migrate from a northern climate to an area closer to the equator or in the opposite direction, your chance of acquiring M.S. is determined pretty much by where you resided prior to age fifteen, suggesting that there was an exposure just before this period of life though the disease may not appear until years later. For example, people who have migrated to Israel from northern Europe have a different likelihood of acquiring the disease than if they migrated to Israel from Africa. Their chance of acquiring the disease statistically relates to where they lived before age fifteen.

Certain black people in Africa and in the Caribbean as well as some Japanese have a kind of partial paraplegia that is not M.S., but is caused by a herpes virus known as HTLV-I. This virus *has no known connection* with the AIDS virus. Some patients with multiple sclerosis also have the HTLV-I virus, as determined by both antigens and antibodies in their blood or spinal fluid.

Medical Treatment and Management of Multiple Sclerosis

The surest sign that there is no cure for multiple sclerosis at the present time is the long list of available treatments currently in use. Many drugs claimed to be of value in the past have been thrown out, while others are undergoing study for the future in centers dedicated to clinical trials of new drugs. This is where the excitement is, because the past decade has been marked by an extraordinary dedication of time and research funds to finding a specific treatment for this unpredictable disease. And we are much closer than ever before to our goal.

This section may be used as an educational reference. Relevant portions may be read for quick informational purposes, but consult your doctor for advice on what applies to your case.

ANTIVIRAL AGENTS

Interferon beta is the first drug available for treatment that alters the underlying course of M.S. It is derived from a protein that has been modified by genetic engineering in bacteria. This basic substance is produced in response to a viral infection and is classified currently as both an antiviral agent and an immune system modulator. Since post-viral infection and impairment of immunological mechanisms have both been incriminated in multiple sclerosis, it should come as no surprise that the Food and Drug Administration has approved this drug for relapsing-remitting multiple sclerosis. Marketed under the brand name Betaseron, this drug has been developed by Berlex Laboratories. While the precise mechanism of the drug's action has not been defined yet, it has been postulated that this antiviral compound may combat fundamental immune abnormalities that contribute to exacerbations of M.S.

In the first clinical trials, 372 patients with the relapsing-remitting form of the disease who could still walk were treated over a course of three years. Approximately one third of the patients received high-dose interferon beta; another one third got a lower dose of the drug and the last third received a placebo. Each treatment was administered under the skin by subcutaneous injection every other day throughout the study. Patients were monitored closely and the following findings were published in the April 1993 edition of *Neurology*.

The high-dose-treated people did far better than the low-dose or placebo groups. They had fewer attacks annually, more exacerbation-free time, milder attacks when they did occur, and fewer patient days in hospitals. Very importantly, there was a significant reduction in the activity of the disease as measured by the number and size of lesions in MRI scans which were followed at frequent intervals.

These data indicate that interferon beta is the first scientifically accepted treatment which alters the natural course of mild to moderate relapsing-remitting M.S. It does not, however, make any statement regarding its potential success or failure in other forms of the disease such as progressive, step-wise, or stable cases.

The common side effects of interferon beta include flu-like symptoms, such as fatigue, chills, fever, and muscle aching, all of which usually decrease over the course of a year. Local inflammatory reactions at the injection site or some relatively minor liver and immune function laboratory abnormalities were also noted in some cases.

The drug is not recommended yet for all people with M.S. and, due to limitations of availability, in the first year or two of production, the drug is being distributed by Berlex Laboratories on the basis of a national lottery, based on lists of potentially treatable candidates provided by their physicians across the country. A spokesman for the Berlex company has reported on National Public Radio that the company expects to have enough of the drug available within two years to cover all M.S. patients who need it.

This drug is *not* a cure-all for M.S., nor is it designed for everyone with this condition, but it does appear that the natural history of M.S. can now be favorably altered with reasonable safety in appropriately selected cases. While it is not yet the beginning of the end of M.S., it probably is at least the end of the beginning.

It is important to distinguish interferon beta from interferon gamma, which should *not* be used because it is known to cause worsening of multiple sclerosis. A third form, interferon alpha, has a weak effect in reducing the number of attacks, but unfortunately does not seem to alter the progression of M.S. The alpha form, therefore, is still regarded as experimental.

Amantadine (Symmetrel), another antiviral drug, was originally chemically synthesized to prevent infection by the influenza type A virus and is a relatively safe product. We currently use it primarily to reduce excessive fatigability in M.S. patients. Amantadine may produce significantly fewer relapses in treated patients compared to controls too, but no effect on disability levels has been clearly demonstrated. This is the reason it is used principally as a symptomatic treatment of fatigue in M.S. patients.

IMMUNOSUPPRESSANT TREATMENTS

Treatments that dampen the immune system deserve emphasis, because they have important potential in the treatment of M.S. While the immune system is complex, the basic units are two types of white blood cells. The larger of these cells are called macrophages (from the Greek "big eaters") which surround and consume debris. They also release a substance, termed a plasminogen activator, which is capable of destroying myelin. Macrophages also release substances known as prostaglandins which promote inflammation and alter immune functions, in both positive and negative ways.

The second type of white blood cells are known as lymphocytes, which, in turn, consist of two basic types. B lymphocytes are made in the bone marrow and produce antibodies. T lymphocytes, on the other hand, are produced mainly by the thymus gland in the chest. T lymphocytes can be divided into several subtypes that are of great importance to our understanding of how the disease becomes aggravated and how, therefore, it may be treated.

When a foreign substance called an antigen enters the environment of the body, T lymphocytes become activated. T-helper cells appear in greater number during attacks. T-killer cells may also appear on the scene, but as the exacerbation begins to turn into a remission with clearing of the attack phase, there is a measurable increase in the number of T-suppressor lymphocytes. So the goal of treatment is to increase the number of "good guys" (T-suppressor cells) and to reduce the population of the "bad guys" (T-helper and T-killer cells).

Many B lymphocytes are found in and around the plaques of M.S. patients, but the type of lymphocyte predominating in the cerebral spinal fluid of M.S. patients is the T lymphocyte. The worse the attack, the more T-helper cells are found circulating there.

With that brief background about immune mechanisms, let's take a look at some of the available immunosuppressant treatments currently being studied experimentally or used in clinical situations. We may assume for the purposes of this discussion that the ultimate purpose of immunosuppressive treatment is to try to halt the progression of M.S. by suppressing abnormal responses in the immune system. We may also assume that certain aspects of our present information on treatment will change before this book goes to press.

Azathioprine (Imuran) may kill certain lymphocytes or reduce their formation. There is no immediate benefit in most treated folks, but a modest dampening effect over a longer period of time has been found in certain cases. Because of potentially serious side effects, however, azathioprine is currently reserved primarily for severe progressive cases and has very limited usefulness due to significant risk factors. It should only be considered where the potential risks of azathioprine outweigh the calculated risks of more severe disability from the disease. In general this product has limited usefulness today for M.S. patients.

Cyclophosphamide (Cytoxan) is an anticancer agent that works because of its immunosuppressant abilities. In other words, it has the capacity to kill lymphocytes. Some controlled studies have suggested that cyclophosphamide will stabilize or halt the progressive form of the disease for approximately two years, but other conflicting reports indicate that this plateau in the progressive course may just be part of the natural course of the illness. Therefore, current thinking is that cyclophosphamide should be reserved for progressive cases that have failed to respond to other, safer treatments.

Another reason this agent is generally reserved for actively progessive and severe cases is because of its potential toxicity. Transient bone marrow suppression occurs, reducing the number of white blood cells temporarily, which lowers the body's resistance to infection. Alopecia (hair loss) is another temporary side effect, but hair usually grows back to its original thickness or thicker within six months. Nausea, vomiting, and the risk of superimposed infection while immunosuppressed are often risk factors to keep in mind. Cyclophosphamide is commonly given in conjunction with a steroid drug such as ACTH.

Cyclosporine A selectively holds back the T-helper lymphocytes and probably works better than placebo in treated patients, but it has potential serious side effects. Because of its high cost and risk of adverse effects, the drug is regarded as investigational. It has not prevented exacerbations or halted progression of M.S. consistently, but one cooperative U.S. study in over 400 patients demonstrated a statistically significant slowing of progression. The data on this drug is still incomplete.

Copolymer I (Cop-I) consists of a protein chain of four amino acids that is a synthetic analogue resembling the myelin basic protein molecule (MBP). This drug is still being investigated and is not yet well enough understood for widespread use in treating the exacerbating-remitting form of M.S., but controlled studies have demonstrated a tendency for it to reduce the number of exacerbations. In the laboratory MBP will protect animals from developing experimental allergic encephalomyelitis (EAE), the laboratory model of multiple sclerosis, if the animals are first immunized with it. MBP may act as a desensitizing vaccine, because treated experimental animals do not develop EAE when they are challenged with the antigen responsible for that disease.

Plasmapheresis is a very expensive form of treatment. The process consists of removing a patient's blood and separating the liquid plasma from the cells in a centrifuge. Then the plasma, which contains lymphocytes and antibodies, is discarded and replaced by normal plasma. Finally, the reconstituted blood is pumped back into the patient's bloodstream. This cycle is repeated multiple times at designated intervals to constitute one course of treatment.

It is not unusual for plasmapheresis to be offered in conjunction with immunosuppressant drugs in order to try to enhance its potential benefits. Some investigators have found that M.S. patients who received plasma exchanges together with low-dose cyclophosphamide and alternate-day prednisone did better than people treated with sham plasmapheresis plus these same drugs. Unfortunately, other statistical analyses of the data failed to confirm these findings, so there is still controversy even among experts as to whether or not the offending antibodies have been effectively removed or not. In conclusion, this form of therapy may have some benefit and is relatively free of serious side effects, but remains very expensive.

Total lymphoid irradiation consists of radiating lymph nodes throughout the body for five to six weeks in order to reduce their autoimmune responsiveness. In M.S. the lymphocytes that have produced antibodies are attacking one's own self, because of a failure of recognition. Protein factors in myelin may look like a foreign antigen to the antibody, and that could be the crux of the recognition problem.

Total lymphoid irradiation has been demonstrated to be relatively safe in patients with other diseases, such as Hodgkin's disease, but due to the high cost and potential remote risks, its use should be reserved at the present time mainly for investigational studies on the chronic-progressive forms of M.S. The long-term hazards of total lymphoid irradiation include baldness, fatigue, pericarditis or inflammation around the heart, shingles, and other non-specific symptoms.

Monoclonal antibodies have been produced through advances in biotechnology to react only with certain types of lymphocytes. Starting with earlier studies on mouse monoclonal antibodies, we can now produce human monoclonal antibodies. This more precise form, instead of shooting all lymphocytes like a spraying shotgun, is able to very selectively hit targets in a more focused way. Some of the new studies involving monoclonal antibody therapy are quite exciting and hold promise for the future, but not all of the controlled trials with this drug are yet in. With significant potential risks and great expense as remaining concerns, monoclonal antibodies are not generally available at the time this chapter is being written.

TREATMENTS OF NO ESTABLISHED VALUE
OR WITH EXCESSIVE RISKS

Acyclovir (Zovirax) is a helpful antiviral agent for certain conditions caused by the herpes simplex or zoster, but has not been shown to be useful yet as an antiviral drug for M.S. It is relatively free of serious adverse effects in short-term use, but might not be as safe in long-term use.

Chlorambucil (Leukeran) appears to have no place in M.S. from scientific studies.

Colchicine has plausible benefit, significant serious side effects, and is still investigational.

Danazol also has plausible benefit, but is still an investigational product.

Interferon gamma, unlike the beta form, causes exacerbations of the disease.

Levamisole is still investigational and has conflicting evidence for and against its efficacy.

Lomustine and *5-Fluorouracil* are both potentially harmful agents in the M.S. setting.

Methotrexate has been adequately tested and demonstrated to be of no value for the treatment of M.S.

Mitoxantrone (Novatrone) has never been adequately tested for M.S., is regarded as experimental, and carries significant risks.

Thymectomy, or removal of the thymus gland, has been adequately tested and has been shown to be of no value for M.S. patients.

Thymus hormones have no generally accepted scientific value for M.S.

Transfer factor has no place in the treatment of M.S., because no benefits have been demonstrated.

STEROIDS

The steroid drug *ACTH* or, more commonly now, *methylprednisolone,* is still the first line of defense in attacks that do not remit spontaneously. ACTH may be administered intramuscularly in twice-daily doses for periods of ten to fourteen days or injected intravenously in the form of *Cortrosyn* in a solution of glucose and water run in over about five to six hours daily for a similar duration. There has been a recent shift from ACTH to methylprednisolone, which is administered intravenously either in ambulatory care centers or in hospitalized patients over five to seven days of treatment.

Steroids work to reduce inflammation, but probably also have some effect on the immune system by stimulating the adrenal gland to produce more glucocorticoid hormones. These hormones in turn help the body to reduce swelling and inflammation. By acting on T lymphocytes, they have immunosuppressive effects.

Temporary improvement in the conduction of electrical impulses along nerves, even through areas of demyelination, has been demonstrated in the laboratory. Over twenty years ago, a well randomized double-blind, multicenter study demonstrated that the duration of an acute exacerbation could be modestly shortened by about 15 percent with a steroid drug.

It is common practice now for neurologists and other physicians who treat multiple sclerosis to follow a course of intravenous treatment with about one month of every-other-day prednisone therapy. The tapering dose helps to sustain the immunosuppressive effect. The risk of long-term use of steroids is minimized by limiting the course to one month and by administering it on an every-other-day basis.

No one should ever receive long-term steroids for M.S., because of serious risks and lack of benefits. Risk factors of long-term steroids include osteoporosis, pathological fractures of bone, gastrointestinal bleeding, psychoses, cataracts, adrenal insufficiency, and a host of other serious problems nobody wants or needs. Occasionally, very severe progressive M.S. patients have been chronically maintained on *every-other-day* prednisone tablets, but only in selected situations and under close supervision should long-term, alternate-day steroids be considered.

Some people believe that methylprednisolone administered intravenously may work faster and more effectively than ACTH, but it requires close medical supervision and may be contraindicated in certain conditions such as heart disease. Serious reactions with the drug occur, but only rarely.

Injection of the drug directly into the spinal fluid by the so-called intrathecal route is now deemed dangerous and has not proven effective. A number of cases of arachnoiditis have appeared following such injections into the subarachnoid space with a chronic inflammatory reaction resulting in scarring that may be permanent. In summary, short-term, high-dose intravenous steroids are an effective first-line treatment defense for cases of M.S. appropriately selected during attack phases.

SYMPTOMATIC TREATMENT

Though not curative, the selective treatment of specific symptoms may improve the M.S. patient's functioning and, therefore, substantially enhance the quality of life for that person. It should be recalled, when using any treatment for M.S., that the natural history of this disease is to spontaneously remit; therefore, an improvement following the introduction of a new medication should not necessarily imply that the drug is responsible for the benefit. Since getting better may be a natural phenomenon or spontaneous remission, I frequently tell my patients, "You got better in spite of me, not because of me." This phenomenon of spontaneous improvement is one of the key factors which makes the evaluation of drugs for M.S. so difficult. That's why double-blind studies in large populations are necessary to eliminate naturally occurring remissions as factors in improvement, rather than giving the credit for "acts of God" to the pharmaceutical companies. There are few gods in this business.

Fatigue is probably the most common symptom of multiple sclerosis. Its causes are multifactorial. Fatigue may result from normal exertion, but M.S. patients become far more fatigued with less exertion in shorter periods of time compared to other individuals. The coincidence of depression of mood may compound the tendency for fatigue, and may be treated with an anti-depressant agent, but it cannot be assumed that all patients with fatigue are therefore depressed. Thorough assessment requires careful psychological as well as neurological evaluation. See the right kind of doctor for these questions.

Pemoline (Cylert) is a stimulant drug that is not an amphetamine like Ritalin or Dexedrine and has few of their undesirable side effects. Pemoline is also widely used for the treatment of attention deficit disorder in children and adults and of narcolepsy. More than 60 percent of M.S. patients treated with this product show a good benefit.

Unlike amphetamines, there is no tendency for physiological or psychological dependence with pemoline. It usually does *not* produce loss of appetite, weight loss, or insomnia to the extent that amphetamines do. While clinical improvement may take three to four weeks, pemoline, given over adequate periods of time, has been shown to be of substantial value in the treatment of fatigue for M.S. patients.

Amantadine (Symmetrel), introduced originally for treatment of the influenza A virus, was later demonstrated to improve the symptoms of Parkinson's disease by releasing a neurotransmitter called dopamine from nerve endings. Now it is used for the treatment of M.S. too. It usually has no serious side effects, though the drug may cause confusion or hallucinations in the elderly and occasionally causes urinary retention. Its action is to relieve the feeling of chronic fatigue and does so in about 50 percent of treated cases, maybe a little less effectively than pemoline, though each case needs to be individualized. One advantage of amantadine is its relative safety, but further studies need to be carried out to determine if this agent can significantly reduce the number of relapses compared to controls as a study in 1987 claimed. For the time being, its principle use in M.S. is for the management of fatigue.

Neurogenic bladder disorders come in three basic varieties and they are usually due to compromised nerve supply to the bladder in M.S. patients.

1. The atonic bladder is large and baggy like an overstretched balloon. Therefore, it is weak in emptying, causes hesitancy, and predisposes a person to the risk of recurrent bladder and kidney infections.
2. The hypertonic or spastic bladder is small and irritable with a smaller urinary capacity. Accordingly, it

produces symptoms of frequency, urgency, and incontinence of urinary control.

3. A combination of the other two bladder disorders most commonly occurs when there is bladder infection combined with an incoordination between the muscles which contract to empty the bladder and the sphincter muscles which control relaxation at the urethral opening. In this situation, a person may have a large residual urine remaining in the bladder after partial emptying has occurred, thereby predisposing to bladder and kidney infections.

To reduce the risk of urinary infections, all patients with multiple sclerosis should be checked periodically for infection with routine urinalyses and cultures on clean voided specimens, even when there are no urinary symptoms. Many people in this category, who are prone to recurrent infection, are carried on a urinary antiseptic drug such as Bactrim or Mandelamine.

The chance of acquiring urinary infection may be reduced if the urine is made more acid by taking large amounts of vitamin C (ascorbic acid tablets) and cranberry juice. A large residual urine volume may be identified by measuring the residual urine. This is done by a physician with a straight catheter following spontaneous voiding or by examining the bladder for retained IVP dye following a kidney X ray.

Oxybutynin (Ditropan) or *flavoxate (Urispas)* is effective in treating overactive or spastic bladders. Both drugs work directly on the smooth muscle of the bladder to reduce spasm. *Propantheline (Pro-Banthine)* works on the nerve endings of the parasympathetic nervous system and is probably a little less effective in reducing bladder spasms.

Self-catheterization by a sterile technique is advisable for patients with large post-voiding residual urine volumes. This simple procedure can be carried out by a person on oneself. If upper extremities are too weak or incoordinate, a caregiver may be trained to assist.

Bathanechol (Urecholine) is designed to stimulate the parasympathetic nervous system for patients with under-active bladder muscles. It helps to initiate urination and provides more complete emptying of a sluggish bladder.

In the mixed type of bladder disorder, a drug to reduce bladder spasms is often combined with intermittent clean catheterization. The use of an indwelling Foley catheter should be avoided if possible, since its presence inevitably leads to urinary tract infections. Adult diapers or, in males, condom catheters are preferable alternatives to catheters for the incontinent patient.

Chronic constipation is a common problem in weak, disabled M.S. patients, particularly those who fail to consume adequate amounts of fluid. We commonly recommend increasing fluid intake, switching to a high fiber diet, and taking a stool softener such as Peri-Colace and/or Metamucil.

Incontinence of bowel control is uncommon in the management of M.S. When it does occur, it can usually be treated either with a drug for diarrhea or an anticholinergic agent to reduce bowel contractility.

Cold and *heat* are important considerations in the symptomatic management of M.S., because the condition is a heat-labile disorder. Sitting in hot sun or taking a hot bath or shower may worsen symptoms and can be reversed by a cool shower or a plunge in cold water. I have seen a quadriplegic patient treated with a cooling blanket make a spontaneous remission in less than twenty-four hours simply by lowering his body temperature.

Swimming in cool water is excellent therapy
all patients with weakness or stiffness from M.S.
4-Aminopyridine (4-AP) is a chemical which
potassium movement and prolongs the action poten
in nerves. In this way, 4-AP can restore conduction to
nerve fibers where the myelin covering has been damaged. Caution must be exercised, however, because the
drug has the potential to cause convulsions, but usually
only when large doses are used. While 4-AP is largely
an investigational drug, it bears watching as an agent with
considerable potential benefit. A related drug, 3,4-DAP,
is also currently under study for the treatment of M.S.

Spasticity may be treated with a variety of antispastic
agents to improve mobility and walking ability. Antispastic agents work well in people with spastic limbs from
spinal cord involvement, so long as taking away the spasticity doesn't leave the patient feeling weaker by removing
the crutch-like benefit of spasticity.

Baclofen (Lioresal) is generally regarded as the most effective and least toxic agent for alleviating spasticity. It
may improve bladder and bowel control, and is of value
in selected cases with pseudobulbar palsy. The latter condition is uncommon, but consists of involuntary laughter
and crying due to M.S. plaques in descending motor
pathways known as the cortico-bulbar tracts. The drug
doesn't work for everyone, but has a high degree of success in this type of emotional dyscontrol.

Diazepam (Valium), while generally a little less effective
than baclofen, works for some spastic people if baclofen
has caused side effects. It is particularly useful for flexor
or extensor spasms of legs occurring either with or without
pain. Those spasms can be particularly troublesome at
bedtime. A single 5- or 10-mg. dose of diazepam before
going to sleep may reduce nocturnal spasms which oth-

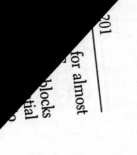

...nia. The prolonged use of di-
...ly advisable, because it leads to
...h medications need to be mon-

...n oral agent which has been
... This drug reduces spasms by
...l cord and has been especially
...of ankle movement known as
... muscle stiffness in M.S. pa-
...been refractory to other antispastic drugs.
One advantage of tizanidine is that it seems to have less
sedative effect than either diazepam or baclofen. It has
been scientifically demonstrated to be an effective agent
and relatively free of serious adverse side effects, even
though it has been less widely used in the United States
than the other two antispastic agents.

Dantrolene (Dantrium) reduces spasticity by acting directly on muscle fibers. Unfortunately, it has the potential
risk of producing serious liver damage or pleural fluid
collections around the lungs. These adverse effects have
limited its usefulness in this country. A small number of
fatal liver failure cases has pushed dantrolene lower on
the list of drugs chosen to treat spasticity.

Ketazolam is similar to diazepam and is just about as
effective in relieving spasticity. Less is known about its
risks, and the possible occurrence of long-term, serious
side effects must be kept in mind.

Surgical manipulations may be considered in severe
cases refractory to medical treatment. By injecting phenol
or alcohol into nerves, or by cutting nerves (neurotomy)
or by cutting nerve roots (rhizotomy), the most severe
spastic or contracted patients may have a better chance
for symptomatic relief of frozen limbs. Muscles or tendons may be cut or tendons transplanted in special cases.

These uncommon procedures are more apt to be done in a chronic rehabilitative hospital setting than in community practice and are designed for severe, intractable situations which have been refractory to medical treatment. The value of this therapy has been scientifically documented, but it carries significant risks, and is expensive.

Diets may be supplemented with linoleic acid or natural oils that contain polyunsaturated fatty acids. The body synthesizes these substances into fatty acids as precursors of myelin in the central nervous system. Various sources of polyunsaturated fatty acids include sunflower seed oil, safflower seed oil, and evening primrose oil. There are conflicting opinions as to whether such a diet really reduces the frequency or severity of M.S. attacks, but some studies have suggested fewer attacks and less disability in people on this kind of diet. Such a diet is safe if supervised by a physician or nutritionist.

Numerous other healthy and fad diets have been proposed. There is a fish-oil diet which has a rather unpleasant fishy taste and conflicting evidence regarding its efficacy. The low-fat diet, while healthy, has not proven to be of significant value in altering the course of M.S. So far, no well-controlled study has shown the effectiveness of the low-fat diet, although it is recommended. There are a host of other diets which have been proposed by both competent and quack diet specialists, but in general a well-balanced diet with generous amounts of polyunsaturated fatty acids and adequate amounts of fiber and water seem to work about as well as anything else on the market today.

Cannabis (Marijuana and its various forms) have no generally accepted scientific basis for use in M.S. therapy, even though some patients report anecdotally that their spasticity improves after smoking marijuana. On the negative side, the long-term use of pot has been shown to impair memory, cognition, and personality, so there are potential serious side effects from the long-term use of tetrahydrocannabinol (THC), the key chemical ingredient in marijuana.

Acupuncture may result in relief from pain or muscle spasms, but it has not been studied scientifically in this country. It is supported by anecdotal observations of Chinese medical practice over centuries. Certainly acupuncture does not get at the underlying disease process, but it may still help to minimize symptoms, especially when elements of pain exist, as it has a kind of anesthetic effect.

There are probably more than *fifty other treatments* for which claims have been made regarding benefit in M.S., but for which there is *absolutely no scientific rationale*. In some, subsequent scientific studies have shown that the drugs were, in fact, dangerous and without any real benefit. Many of these substances have had no controlled study and carry serious risks. Therefore it is important that M.S. patients obtain treatment in a reputable facility from physicians experienced in the management of multiple sclerosis.

M.S. clinics under the auspices of the National Multiple Sclerosis Society usually include at least a neurologist and a nurse or psychology counselor. Access to a urologist for bladder disorders, equipment for performing cystometrograms to measure the pressure dynamics of neurogenic bladders and good laboratory services are also available in most M.S. clinics.

The psychological support of the patient and family is as important as the neurological and medical team. Psychologists for supportive therapy and neuropsychologists for testing memory and cognitive disorders are helpful coaches to address common concerns of M.S. patients and their families.

An appropriate blend of regular physical exercise, as tolerated, and strengthening of the spirit through whatever avenue works in the individual case is standard practice in most clinics dedicated to the treatment of multiple sclerosis. These kind of services can usually be found in a Multiple Sclerosis clinic under the auspices of the National Multiple Sclerosis Society.

Limitations and Risks of Treatment

The doctor should meet with the M.S. patient and his family to explain the natural course of the disease and the potential risks and benefits of the various therapies. Sometimes it may be best to temporize and wait to see if a spontaneous remission will occur. Of course, in some situations it may be important to act quickly, as when visual acuity has been threatened. Remember, more than 50 percent of patients will improve in one year even when not treated. Nonetheless, you should see a physician with expertise in multiple sclerosis to be sure that the diagnosis is accurate and treatment suggestions are reasonable. No treatment can be guaranteed successful in advance of a trial. Dosages need to be adequate, and the method of administering the medicine needs to be controlled. Treatment failure with one drug or one dosage may not necessarily imply failure with other alternatives. Successful treatment may mean a temporary remission for less than one year or a halting of the progression of the disease for two years or longer. There are cases on record of natural remissions that lasted for many years even without treatment.

REHABILITATION

Physical and occupational therapy and an ongoing home exercise program play an important role in conjunction with medical drug therapy. Walking and swimming, maintaining muscle tone, and passive stretching exercises prevent joint contracture and help to maintain a healthier state. Keeping the body moving and turning frequently from side to side prevents the development of bedsores. Bladder care advised by your doctor may prevent recurrent infections, which in turn may prevent new exacerbations or chronic kidney problems from developing. Clean voided urine specimens should be cultured to look for treatable infections.

SUPPORTIVE THERAPY

This treatment comes in many forms. Counselors experienced in the emotional needs of M.S. patients are the ones to seek out. The local chapters of the National M.S. Society may be able to refer you to clinic centers or individuals who have the most experience in your area, whether they are psychologists, social workers, visiting nurses, or physicians. Your state chapter of the National M.S. Society has a wealth of printed material and interested, knowledgeable people who can help you if you simply call them and state your needs.

Evaluating Claims by Investigators, Physicians, and the News Media

A word of caution about "breakthrough" claims and exaggerated reports is necessary. Perhaps there is no other disease that has received more "hype" in the news media than the writings about multiple sclerosis. But you have to look at all claims with a jaundiced eye. Check with your state chapter of the M.S. Society or your doctor to be sure that these "easy cure" claims are not simply inflated facts or quack reports. Even the work of highly respected and cautious investigators may be misquoted in the news media, only to bring about false hopes. At all costs, try to avoid "desperation shots," when no one seems to have a cure for a progressing condition. Stay with highly reputable medical centers and if necessary get a second opinion, but only from respected centers, clinics, or doctors known for their conservative approach to multiple sclerosis. At the same time, be sure you have a primary doctor to take care of your general health in addition to the specialist who manages your neurological condition.

In 1987, the National Multiple Sclerosis Society spent almost $7 million on M.S. research. No one knows when a cure or prevention for this disease will be forthcoming, but we look forward to the day when M.S. will go the way of diphtheria and poliomyelitis, either through the development of immunosuppressant drugs or through the development of a vaccine to wipe this disease from the surface of the earth forever.

SOURCES OF
HELP AND INFORMATION

The resource lists were prepared with the able assistance of Cynthia Zagieboylo, director of Support Services, Massachusetts Chapter, National Multiple Sclerosis Society.

The most helpful organization for people with multiple sclerosis and their families is the National Multiple Sclerosis Society. The Society was founded in 1946 at a time when only two researchers in the country expressed interest in multiple sclerosis research. Since its founding the Society has generated over $100 million in research grants and fellowships.

The goals of the Society are to:

provide service to people with multiple sclerosis and their families;

educate the medical community and general public;

promote research into the cause, prevention, cure, and treatment of the disease.

208

The Society fulfills its mission through the activities of the national organization and nearly one hundred local chapters.

For information on local chapters, write to:
National Multiple Sclerosis Society
733 Third Avenue
New York, NY 10017-3288
(212) 986-3240
(800) 532-7667
FAX (212) 986-7981

National Multiple Sclerosis Society Chapters

Alabama Chapter
3125 Montgomery Highway,
  Suite 303
Birmingham, AL 35209
(205) 879-8881
(800) 373-8881
FAX (205) 870-8726

Alaska Chapter
511 West 41st Avenue,
  Suite 101
Anchorage, AK 99503
(907) 563-1115
(800) 478-1115
FAX (907) 562-6673

Desert Southwest Chapter
P.O. Box 61654
Phoenix, AZ 85082
(602) 277-8459
(800) 737-8459
FAX (602) 966-4049

Arkansas Chapter
1100 North University,
  Suite 255
Evergreen Place
Little Rock, AR 72207
(501) 663-6767
(800) 482-5945
FAX (501) 666-4355

California Chapters
Central California Chapter
770 East Shaw #217
Fresno, CA 93710
(209) 226-2005
(800) 524-7061
FAX (209) 226-2065

Southern California Chapter
230 N. Maryland Avenue,
  Suite 303
Glendale, CA 91206
(818) 247-1175
(800) 243-5767
FAX (818) 247-1364

Orange County Chapter
17752 Mitchell, Suite F
Irvine, CA 92714
(714) 752-1680
(800) 486-MSOC (National)
FAX (714) 833-3104

Northern California Chapter
150 Grand Avenue
Oakland CA 94612
(510) 268-0572
(800) FIGHT-MS
  (344-4867)
FAX (510) 451-8796

Mountain Valley California
  Chapter
2277 Watt Avenue, Suite A
Sacramento, CA 95825
(916) 486-8981
(800) 222-NMSS
FAX (916) 486-1190

San Diego Area Chapter
4715 Viewridge Avenue,
  Suite 150
San Diego, CA 92123
(619) 974-8640
(800) 447-6773
FAX (619) 974-8646

Channel Islands Chapter
3022-A De La Vina
Santa Barbara, CA 93105
(805) 682-8783
(800) 367-9195
FAX (805) 563-1489

Santa Clara County Chapter
2589 Scott Blvd.
Santa Clara, CA 95050
(408) 988-7557
FAX (408) 988-1816

Colorado Chapter
1777 South Harrison,
  Suite 200
Denver, CO 80210
(303) 691-2956
(800) 342-2873
FAX (303) 758-8349

Connecticut Chapters
Western Connecticut
  Chapter
83 East Avenue, Suite 113
Norwalk, CT 06851
(203) 838-1033
FAX (203) 831-5155

Greater Connecticut
  Chapter
1155 Silas Deane Highway
Wethersfield, CT 06109
(203) 721-6001
(800) 233-7617
FAX (203) 721-6007

Delaware Chapter
Two Mill Road, Suite 106
Wilmington, DE 19806
(302) 655-5610
(800) 640-1001
FAX (302) 655-0993

National Capital Chapter
2021 K Street NW,
   Suite 100
Washington, DC 20006
(202) 296-5363
(800) 989-6774
FAX (202) 296-3425

Florida Chapters
South Florida Chapter
5410 NW 33rd Avenue,
   #108
Fort Lauderdale, FL 33309
(305) 731-4224
FAX (305) 739-1398

North Florida Chapter
One San Jose Place, Suite 1
Jacksonville, FL 32257
(904) 262-6767
(800) 752-3944
FAX (904) 292-0890

Central Florida Chapter
3191 Maguire Boulevard,
   Suite 185
Orlando, FL 32803
(407) 896-3873
FAX (407) 898-6736

Florida Gulf Coast Chapter
5420 Bay Center Drive,
   Suite 118
Tampa, FL 33609
(813) 287-2939
(800) 922-0170
FAX (813) 286-9576

Georgia Chapter
1100 Circle 75 Parkway,
   Suite 630
Atlanta, GA 30339
(404) 984-9080
(800) 822-3379
FAX (404) 984-9352

Hawaiian Islands Chapter
245 North Kukui Street,
   #104
Honolulu, HI 96817
(808) 531-4127
FAX (808) 538-3503

Idaho Chapter
6901 Emerald, Suite 203
Boise, ID 83704
(208) 322-6721
(800) 834-2006
FAX (208) 322-6210 (Please
   call before faxing)

*Chicago-Greater Illinois
   Chapter*
600 South Federal Street,
   Suite 204
Chicago, IL 60605
(312) 922-8000
(800) 922-0484
FAX (312) 922-2752

Indiana State Chapter
615 North Alabama Street,
   Room 318
Indianapolis, IN 46204
(317) 634-8796
(800) 762-1209
FAX (317) 686-0617

Iowa Chapter
2400 86th Street, Suite 29
Des Moines, IA 50322
(515) 270-6337
(800) 798-6677
FAX (515) 270-0337

Kansas Chapters
Mid-America Chapter
P.O. Box 2292
Shawnee Mission, KS 66201
(913) 432-3926
(800) 745-3148
FAX (913) 432-6912

South Central and West
   Kansas Chapter
250 South Laura
Wichita, KS 67211
(316) 264-1333

Kentucky Chapter
Kosair Charities Centre
982 Eastern Parkway
Louisville, KY 40217
(502) 636-1700
(800) 873-6367
FAX (502) 636-2638

Louisiana Chapter
3616 South I-10 Service
   Road, Suite 101
Metairie, LA 70001
(504) 832-4013
(800) 346-7323
FAX (504) 831-7188

Maine Chapter
P.O. Box 8730
Portland, ME 04104
(207) 761-5815
(800) 639-1330
FAX (207) 761-5817

Maryland Chapter
1055 Taylor Avenue,
   Suite 201
Towson, MD 21286
(410) 821-8626
FAX (410) 821-8030

Massachusetts Chapter
400-1 Totten Pond Road
Waltham, MA 02154
(617) 890-4990
FAX (617) 890-2089

Michigan Chapter
26111 Evergreen, Suite 100
Southfield, MI 48076
(313) 350-0020
(800) 2-HELP-MS
   (243-5767)
FAX (313) 350-0029

Minnesota North Star
   Chapter
2344 Nicollet Avenue
Minneapolis, MN 55404
(612) 870-1500
(800) 582-5296 (National)
FAX (612) 870-0265

Mississippi Chapter
6055 Highway 18 South
Jackson, MS 39209
(601) 922-7979
(800) 734-6092
FAX (601) 922-8048

Gateway Area Chapter
915 Olive Street, Suite 310
Saint Louis, MO 63101
(314) 241-8285
(800) 628-1753
FAX (314) 241-8836

Montana Chapter
1601 2nd Avenue North
Great Falls, MT 59401
(406) 452-9529
(800) 423-1820
FAX (406) 452-4315

Midlands Chapter
Community Health Plaza
7101 Newport Avenue,
    Suite 203
Omaha, NE 68152
(800) 755-3959
FAX (402) 572-3002

Great Basin Sierra Chapter
3100 Mill Street, Suite 115
Reno, NV 89502
(702) 329-7180
(800) 800-9295
FAX (702) 329-7256

New Hampshire Chapter
50 Bridge Street, Suite 262
Manchester, NH 03101
(603) 623-3501
(800) 639-3501
FAX (603) 623-4205

New Jersey Chapters
Mid-Jersey Chapter
801 Belmar Plaza
Belmar, NJ 07719
(908) 681-2322
FAX (908) 681-2341

Northern New Jersey
    Chapter
14 Ridgedale Avenue,
    Suite 101
Cedar Knolls, NJ 07927
(201) 984-6667
FAX (201) 984-5658

Bergen-Passaic Counties
    Chapter
P.O. Box 348
730 River Road, 2nd Floor
New Milford, NJ 07646
(201) 967-5599

Rio Grande Chapter
2021 Girard SE, Suite 112
Albuquerque, NM 87106
(505) 842-6767
(800) 224-8883
FAX (505) 842-0055

New York Chapters
Capital District Chapter
324 Broadway, 4th Floor
Albany, NY 12207
(518) 427-0421
(800) 922-9120
FAX (518) 427-0426

South Central New York
  Chapter
32 West State Street,
  1st Floor
Binghamton, NY 13901
(607) 724-5464
(800) 640-9232

Western New York/
  Northwestern
  Pennsylvania Chapter
2060 Sheridan Drive
Buffalo, NY 14223
(716) 875-7710
(800) 765-4677
FAX (716) 875-7786

Long Island Chapter
200 Parkway Drive South,
  Suite 101
Hauppauge, NY 11788
(516) 864-8337
FAX (516) 864-8342

Southern New York Chapter
11 Skyline Drive
Hawthorne, NY 10532
(914) 345-3500
FAX (914) 345-3504

New York City Chapter
30 West 26th Street,
  9th Floor
New York, NY 10010
(212) 463-7787
FAX (212) 989-4362

Rochester Area Chapter
1000 Elmwood Avenue
Rochester, NY 14620
(716) 271-0801
FAX (716) 442-7573

Upstate New York Chapter
404 Oak Street
Syracuse, NY 13203
(315) 422-1447
FAX (315) 422-1603

North Carolina Chapters
Greater Carolinas Chapter
1515 Mockingbird Lane,
  Suite 1000
Charlotte, NC 28209
(704) 525-2955
(800) 477-2955
FAX (704) 527-0406

Central North Carolina
  Chapter
2302 West Meadowview
  Road, Suite 120
Greensboro, NC 27407
(919) 299-4136
FAX (919) 855-3039

Eastern North Carolina
   Chapter
3725 National Drive,
   Suite 115
Raleigh, NC 27612
(919) 781-0676
FAX (919) 781-1042

Mid-Ohio Chapter
1550 Old Henderson Road,
   W-101
Columbus, OH 43220
(614) 459-2220
(800) 522-6655
FAX (614) 459-2929

Dakota Chapter
2801 Main Avenue
Fargo, ND 58103
(701) 235-2678
(800) 437-5844
FAX (701) 235-6358

Western Ohio Chapter
The Woolpert Bldg.
409 East Monument,
   Suite 101
Dayton, OH 45402
(513) 461-5253
FAX (513) 461-3500

Ohio Chapters
Southwest Ohio/Northern
   Kentucky Chapter
The Park Lane Apartments
4201 Victory Parkway, #115
Cincinnati, OH 45229
(513) 281-5200
FAX (513) 281-5162

Northwest Ohio Chapter
415 Tomahawk Drive
Maumee, OH 43537
(419) 897-9533
(800) 368-7459
FAX (419) 897-9733

Northeast Ohio Chapter
The Hanna Building
1422 Euclid Avenue,
   Suite 333
Cleveland, OH 44115
(216) 696-8220
(Clients call collect)
FAX (216) 696-2817

Oklahoma Chapter
Building #7
4606 East 67th Street,
   Suite 201
Tulsa, OK 74136
(918) 488-0882
(800) 777-7814
FAX (918) 488-0913

Oregon Chapter
5901 SW Macadam,
 Suite 100
Portland, OR 97201
(503) 223-9511
(800) 422-3042
FAX (503) 223-2912

Pennsylvania Chapters
Central Pennsylvania
 Chapter
2209 Forest Hills Drive,
 #18
Harrisburg, PA 17112
(717) 652-2108
(800) 227-2108
FAX (717) 652-2590

Lancaster County Chapter
117-D South West End
 Avenue
Lancaster, PA 17603
(717) 397-1481
FAX (717) 393-4030 (When
 sending a fax, please mark
 it clearly to the chapter's
 attention)

Greater Delaware Valley
 Chapter
117 South 17th Street,
 Room 500
Philadelphia, PA 19103
(215) 963-0200
(800) 445-2453
FAX (215) 963-0335

Allegheny District Chapter
1040 Fifth Avenue,
 2nd Floor
Pittsburgh, PA 15219
(412) 261-6347
(800) 544-5250
FAX (412) 232-1461

Puerto Rico Chapter
P.O. Box 29085
San Juan, PR 00929
(809) 763-0303
FAX (809) 764-7312

Rhode Island Chapter
535 Centerville Road
Warwick, RI 02886
(401) 738-8383
FAX (401) 738-8469

South Carolina Chapter
2711 Middleburg Drive,
 Suite 105
Columbia, SC 29204
(803) 799-7848
(800) 922-7591
FAX (803) 798-3825

Tennessee Chapters
Setenga Chapter
P.O. Box 3331
Chattanooga, TN 37404
(615) 624-2064
(800) 523-7088
FAX (615) 622-8737

Mid-South Chapter
755 Crossover Lane
Building A, Suite 101
Memphis, TN 38117
(901) 763-3601
(800) 631-7712
FAX (901) 767-9625

Middle Tennessee Chapter
2200 21st Avenue South,
  Suite 307
Nashville, TN 37212
(615) 269-9055
FAX (615) 269-9470 (When
  sending a fax, please mark
  it clearly to the chapter's
  attention)

Texas Chapters
Panhandle Chapter
715 South Lamar
Amarillo, TX 79106
(806) 372-4429
FAX (806) 372-6421

North Texas Chapter
8214 Westchester Drive,
  Suite 600
Dallas, TX 75225
(214) 373-1400
FAX (214) 373-7200

Tri-Cities of Texas Chapter
6001 Bridge Street,
  Suite 107
Fort Worth, TX 76112
(817) 496-4475
(800) 833-6178
FAX (817) 496-1277

Southeast Texas Chapter
2211 Norfolk, Suite 825
Houston, TX 77098
(713) 526-8967
(800) 323-4873
FAX (713) 526-4049

West Texas Chapter
P.O. Box 4636
Midland, TX 79704
(915) 699-7787
FAX (915) 699-6381

South Texas Chapter
140 Heimer, #195
San Antonio, TX 78232
(210) 494-5531
(800) 683-1627
FAX (210) 494-5545 (please
  call before faxing!)

Utah State Chapter
525 South 300 West
Salt Lake City, UT 84101
(801) 575-8500
(800) 527-8116
FAX (801) 575-8514

Vermont Chapter
Champlain Mill #42
1 Main Street
Winooski, VT 05404
(802) 655-3666

Virginia Chapters
Blue Ridge Chapter
P.O. Box 6808
Charlottesville, VA 22906
(804) 971-8010
(800) 451-0373
FAX (804) 979-4475

Central Virginia Chapter
5001 West Broad Street,
  Suite 220
Richmond, VA 23230
(804) 282-2358
(800) 487-4677
FAX (804) 282-2380

Hampton Roads Chapter
405 South Parliament Drive,
  Suite 105
Virginia Beach, VA 23462
(804) 490-9627 (Southside)
(804) 872-8454 (Peninsula area)
FAX (804) 490-1617

Washington Chapters
Western Washington
  Chapter
192 Nickerson Street,
  Suite 100
Seattle, WA 98109
(206) 284-4236
FAX (206) 284-4972

Inland Northwest Chapter
East 818 Sharp
Spokane, WA 99202
(509) 482-2022
FAX (509) 483-1077

Southwest Washington
  Chapter
6315 South 19th Street
Tacoma, WA 98466
(206) 565-7555

Central Washington Chapter
P.O. Box 1093
Yakima, WA 98907
(509) 248-2350
(800) 288-5256
FAX (509) 248-2352 (When
  sending a fax, please mark
  it clearly to the chapter's
  attention)

West Virginia Chapter
P.O. Box 3064
Charleston, WV 25331
(800) 628-5645
FAX (304) 925-6989

Wisconsin Chapter
W223 N608 Saratoga Drive
Waukesha, WI 53186
(414) 547-8999
(800) 242-3358
FAX (414) 547-4440

Wyoming Chapter
P.O. Box 556
Casper, WY 82602
(307) 234-2340
(800) 367-1491

National Multiple Sclerosis Society Training and Resource Center
116 Inverness Drive East, Suite 205
Englewood, CO 80112
(303) 790-7929
FAX (303) 790-8044

Canadian Chapter
Multiple Sclerosis Society of Canada
130 Bloor Street, W, Suite 700
Toronto, Ontario M5S 1S5

Other agencies that may be helpful to individuals with multiple sclerosis and their families include:

American Coalition of Citizens with Disabilities (ACCD)
1200 15th Street, NW, Suite 201
Washington, DC 20005

American Foundation for the Blind
15 West 16th Street
New York, NY 10111

American Occupational Therapy Association
1383 Picard Drive
P.O. Box 1725
Rockville, MD 20850

American Physical Therapy Association
1156 15th Street, NW
Washington, DC 20005

Disabled American Veterans
P.O. Box 14301
Cincinnati, OH 45214

Foundation for Hospice and Home Care
519 C Street, NE
Washington, DC 20002

National Association of the Physically Handicapped
2810 Terrace Road, SE
Washington, DC 20020

National Easter Society
2023 West Ogden
Chicago, IL 60612

National Rehabilitation
   Information Center
4407 8th Street, NE
Washington, DC 20017

Paralyzed Veterans of
   America
801 18th Street, NW
Washington, DC 20006

President's Committee on
   Employment of the
   Handicapped
Washington, DC 20036

Veterans Administration
810 Vermont Avenue, NW
Washington, DC 20420

In addition to national organizations, there are many resources that may be available in your state or community. They include:

Commissions on Handicapped Affairs
Department of Mental Health
Department of Public Welfare
Department of Social Services
Office for the Blind
Office for Elder Affairs
Office of Handicapped Affairs
Office of Vocational Rehabilitation
Public Housing Authority
Social Security Administration
Visiting Community Nurse Association

Companies that provide adaptive equipment—ambulatory aids, bathroom and toilet aids, dressing and grooming aids, exercise and recreation equipment, wheelchair equipment—to assist individuals with multiple sclerosis include (ask for catalogs):

Access to Independence
1954 East Washington
  Avenue
Madison, WI 53704
(608) 251-7575
(Publications to increase
  independence of disabled)

Activeaid, Inc.
P.O. Box 359
Redwood Falls, MN
  56283-0359
(800) 533-5330
(Bathroom, Toilet,
  wheelchair aids)

Carex
39 Tompkins Point Road
P.O. Box 20260A
Newark, NJ 07101
(201) 824-7637
(Adaptive equipment and
  aids)

CLEO, Inc.
3597 Mayfield Road
Cleveland, OH 44121
(216) 382-9700
(Adaptive and exercise
  equipment and aids)

Enrichments
P.O. Box 579
Hinsdale, IL 60521
(800) 323-5547
(Products to help people
  bathe, eat, read, dress)

Exceptionally Yours, Inc.
60 Joseph Road
P.O. Box 3246
Framingham, MA 01701
(617) 877-9757
(adapted clothing)

Fleetwood
P.O. Box 1259
Holland, MI 49422
(800) 257-6390
(adapted furniture,
  wheelchairs, and aids)

Fred Sammons, Inc.
145 Tower Drive
Burr Ridge, IL 60521
(800) 322-5547
(Self-help aids for hygiene
  and dressing)

Health Equipment, Inc.
P.O. Box 90463
San Diego, CA 92109
(619) 273-5394
Adapted furniture,
  wheelchairs, and aids)

International Healthcare
  Products, Inc.
P.O. Box 4180
Long Grove, IL 60047
(800) 423-7886
(Portable bath lift)

Maddak, Inc.
Pequannock, NJ 07440
(201) 694-0500
(Ableware collection
  for independent
  living)

Ortho-Kinetics, Inc.
P.O. Box 1647
Waukesha, WI 53187
(800) 558-7786
(Complete line of mobility
  products)

Prentke Romich Co.
1022 Heyl Road
Wooster, OH 44691
(800) 642-8255
(Computer access devices for
  disabled persons)

Rusko Writing Company,
  Inc.
P.O. Box 121
Crawfordsville, IN 47933
(317) 362-8914
(Stetro pen and pencil grips)

Sports 'n Spokes
5201 North 19th Avenue,
  Suite 111
Phoenix, AZ 85015
(602) 246-9426
(Magazine devoted to
  wheelchair sports and
  recreation)

Ultramatic Sleep of
  America, Inc.
2045 Niagara Falls
  Boulevard, Unit 5
Niagara Falls, NY 14304
(716) 297-7764
(Electric adjustable beds)

Walker Devices, Inc.
Truman Street
Norwalk, CT 06850
(203) 847-5412
(Mobility devices)

FURTHER READING

There are many books, manuals, and pamphlets that can be very useful to people with multiple sclerosis and their families. Among those published by the National Multiple Sclerosis Society and available from them or your local chapter are:

Emotional Aspects of MS, by Floyd Davis, M.D.

Living with MS: A Practical Guide, edited by Lynn Wasserman.

Maximizing Your Health: A Program of Graded Exercises and Meditation for Persons with Multiple Sclerosis, edited by Robert Buxbaum, M.D., and Debra Frankel, M.S., O.T.R.

Mental Health & MS, by Molly Harrower.

Plaintalk: A Booklet About Multiple Sclerosis for Family Members, by Sarah L. Minden, M.D., and Debra Frankel, M.S., O.T.R.

Sexuality & Multiple Sclerosis, by Michael Barrett, Ph.D., M.S. Society of Canada.

Someone You Know Has Multiple Sclerosis: A Book for Families, by Patricia Dick, et al. (designed for eight- to twelve-year-olds).

Helpful books on multiple sclerosis include:

Living Well with MS: A Guide for Patient, Caregiver, and Family, by David L. Carroll and Jon Dudley Dorman, M.D. (New York: HarperCollins, 1993). Practical manual that includes exercise suggestions.

Mastering Multiple Sclerosis, 2nd edition, by John K. Wolf, M.D. (Rutland, Vt: Academy Books, 1987). A 400-page handbook for individuals with M.S. and their families.

The Multiple Sclerosis Diet Book, by J. Swank, M.D., Ph.D., and Barbara Dugan (Garden City, N.Y.: Doubleday, 1987). Good, nutritious low-fat recipes.

Multiple Sclerosis: A Guide for Patients and Their Families, 2nd edition, by Labe Scheinberg, M.D. (New York: Raven Press, 1987). Practical manual with emphasis on enhancing an M.S. person's quality of life.

Multiple Sclerosis: Your Legal Rights, by Lanny Perkins, Esq., and Sara Perkins, Esq. (New York: Demos Publications, 1987). A valuable guidebook to assist people with legal, insurance, Social Security, employment, and other choices and rights.

The Pursuit of Hope, by Miriam Ottenberg (New York: Rawson, Wade, 1978). A beautifully written classic that provides encouragement and realism.

Symptom Management in Multiple Sclerosis, by Randall T. Shapiro, M.D. (New York: Demos Publications, 1987). A manual that focuses on management of specific symptoms through medication and rehabilitation.

Other books that may be helpful include:

Access to the World—A Travel Guide for the Handicapped, by Louise Weiss (New York: Henry Holt & Co., 1986).

Anatomy of an Illness, by Norman Cousins (New York: W. W. Norton, 1979).

Feeling Good—The New Mood Therapy, by David Burns, M.D. (New York: Signet Books, New American Library, 1981).

A Guide for the Disabled Traveler, by Frances Barish (New York: Simon & Schuster, 1984).

Getting Well Again, by O. Carl Simonton, M.D., et al. (New York: Bantam Books, 1984).

A Handbook for the Disabled, by Suzanne Lunt (New York: Charles Scribner's Sons, 1982).

Living with Chronic Illness: Days of Patience and Passion, by Cheri Register (New York: The Free Press, 1987).

Love, Medicine & Miracles, by Bernie Siegel, M.D. (New York: Harper & Row, 1986).

Reach for Fitness, by Richard Simmons (New York: Warner Books, 1986).

The Relaxation Response, by Herbert Benson, M.D. (New York: Avon Books, 1975).

We Are Not Alone: Learning to Live with Chronic Illness, by Sefra Kobrin Pitzele (New York: Workman Publishing, 1986).

When Bad Things Happen to Good People, by Harold Kushner (New York: Avon Books, 1981).

INDEX

227